D1446475

Medicine & Society
In America

Medicine & Society In America

Advisory Editor

Charles E. Rosenberg
Professor of History
University of Pennsylvania

Sex in Education;

OR,

A Fair Chance for the Girls

BY

EDWARD H. CLARKE, M.D.

*A*RNO *P*RESS & *T*HE *N*EW *Y*ORK *T*IMES

New York   1972

Reprint Edition 1972 by Arno Press Inc.

Reprinted from a copy in
The University of Illinois Library

LC# 74-180566
ISBN 0-405-03943-3

Medicine and Society in America
ISBN for complete set: 0-405-03930-1
See last pages of this volume for titles.

Manufactured in the United States of America

Sex in Education;

OR,

A FAIR CHANCE FOR THE GIRLS.

BY

EDWARD H. CLARKE, M.D.,

MEMBER OF THE MASSACHUSETTS MEDICAL SOCIETY; FELLOW OF
THE AMERICAN ACADEMY OF ARTS AND SCIENCES;
LATE PROFESSOR OF MATERIA MEDICA
IN HARVARD COLLEGE,
ETC., ETC.

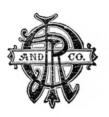

BOSTON:
JAMES R. OSGOOD AND COMPANY,
(LATE TICKNOR & FIELDS, AND FIELDS, OSGOOD, & CO.)
1873.

BOSTON :

STEREOTYPED AND PRINTED BY RAND, AVERY, & CO.

"An American female constitution, which collapses just in the middle third of life, and comes out vulcanized India-rubber, if it happen to live through the period when health and strength are most wanted."

OLIVER WENDELL HOLMES: *Autocrat of the Breakfast Table.*

"He reverenced and upheld, in every form in which it came before him, *womanhood.* . . . What a woman should demand is respect for her as she is a woman. Let her first lesson be, with sweet Susan Winstanley, to *reverence her sex.*"

CHARLES LAMB: *Essays of Elia.*

"We trust that the time now approaches when man's condition shall be progressively improved by the force of reason and truth, when the brute part of nature shall be crushed, that the god-like spirit may unfold."

GUIZOT: *History of Civilization,* I., 34.

CONTENTS.

PREFACE.

————

ABOUT a year ago the author was honored by
an invitation to address the New-England Women's Club in Boston. He accepted the invitation, and selected for his subject the relation of
sex to the education of women. The essay excited an unexpected amount of discussion. Brief
reports of it found their way into the public jour-
nals. Teachers and others interested in the education of girls, in different parts of the country,
who read these reports, or heard of them, made inquiry, by letter or otherwise, respecting it. Various
and conflicting criticisms were passed upon it. This
manifestation of interest in a brief and unstudied
lecture to a small club appeared to the author to
indicate a general appreciation of the importance
of the theme he had chosen, compelled him to
review carefully the statements he had made, and

has emboldened him to think that their publication in a more comprehensive form, with added physiological details and clinical illustrations, might contribute something, however little, to the cause of sound education. Moreover, his own conviction, not only of the importance of the subject, but of the soundness of the conclusions he has reached, and of the necessity of bringing physiological facts and laws prominently to the notice of all who are interested in education, conspires with the interest excited by the theme of his lecture to justify him in presenting these pages to the public. The leisure of his last professional vacation has been devoted to their preparation. The original address, with the exception of a few verbal alterations, is incorporated into them.

Great plainness of speech will be observed throughout this essay. The nature of the subject it discusses, the general misapprehension both of the strong and weak points in the physiology of the woman question, and the ignorance displayed by many, of what the co-education of the sexes really means, all forbid that ambiguity of language or euphemism of expression should be employed in the discussion. The subject is treated solely from the standpoint of physiology. Technical terms have been employed, only where their use is more exact or less offensive than common ones.

If the publication of this brief memoir does nothing more than excite discussion and stimulate investigation with regard to a matter of such vital moment to the nation as the relation of sex to education, the author will be amply repaid for the time and labor of its preparation. No one can appreciate more than he its imperfections. Notwithstanding these, he hopes a little good may be extracted from it, and so commends it to the consideration of all who desire the *best* education of the sexes.

Boston, 18 Arlington Street, October, 1873.

PREFACE TO SECOND EDITION.

THE demand for a second edition of this book in little more than a week after the publication of the first, indicates the interest which the public take in the relation of Sex to Education, and justifies the author in appealing to physiology and pathology for light upon the vexed question of the appropriate education of girls. Excepting a few verbal alterations, and the correction of a few typographical errors, there is no difference between this edition and the first. The author would have been glad to add to this edition a section upon the relation of sex to women's work in life, after their technical education is completed, but has not had time to do so.

BOSTON, 18 ARLINGTON STREET,
Nov. 3, 1873.

NOTE TO THE FIFTH EDITION.

THE attention of the reader is called to the definition of "education" on the twentieth page. It is there stated, that, throughout this essay, education is not used in the limited sense of mental or intellectual training alone, but as comprehending the whole manner of life, physical and psychical, during the educational period; that is, following Worcester's comprehensive definition, as comprehending instruction, discipline, manners, and habits. This, of course, includes home-life and social life, as well as school-life; balls and parties, as well as books and recitations; walking and riding, as much as studying and sewing. When a remission or intermission is necessary, the parent must decide what part of education shall be remitted or omitted, — the walk, the ball, the school, the party, or all of these. None can doubt which will interfere most with Nature's laws, — four hours' dancing, or four hours' studying. These remarks may be unnecessary. They are made because some who have noticed this essay have spoken of it as if it treated only of the school, and seem to have forgotten the just and comprehensive signification in which education is used throughout this memoir. Moreover, it may be well to remind the reader, even at the risk of casting a reflection upon his intelligence, that, in these pages, the relation of sex to mature life is not discussed, except in a few passages, in which the large capacities and great power of woman are alluded to, provided the epoch of development is physiologically guided.

SEX IN EDUCATION.

PART I.

INTRODUCTORY.

"Is there any thing better in a State than that both women and men be rendered the very best? There is not." — PLATO.

IT is idle to say that what is right for man is wrong for woman. Pure reason, abstract right and wrong, have nothing to do with sex: they neither recognize nor know it. They teach that what is right or wrong for man is equally right and wrong for woman. Both sexes are bound by the same code of morals; both are amenable to the same divine law. Both have a right to do the best they can; or, to speak more justly, both should feel the duty, and have the opportunity, to do their

best. Each must justify its existence by be-
coming a complete development of manhood
and womanhood; and each should refuse
whatever limits or dwarfs that development.

The problem of woman's sphere, to use the
modern phrase, is not to be solved by apply-
ing to it abstract principles of right and
wrong. Its solution must be obtained from
physiology, not from ethics or metaphysics.
The question must be submitted to Agassiz
and Huxley, not to Kant or Calvin, to Church
or Pope. Without denying the self-evident
proposition, that whatever a woman can do, she
has a right to do, the question at once arises,
What can she do? And this includes the further question, What can she best do? A girl
can hold a plough, and ply a needle, after a
fashion. If she can do both better than a man,
she ought to be both farmer and seamstress;
but if, on the whole, her husband can hold
best the plough, and she ply best the needle,
they should divide the labor. He should be
master of the plough, and she mistress of the
loom. The *quæstio vexata* of woman's sphere

will be decided by her organization. This limits her power, and reveals her divinely-appointed tasks, just as man's organization limits his power, and reveals his work. In the development of the organization is to be found the way of strength and power for both sexes. Limitation or abortion of development leads both to weakness and failure.

Neither is there any such thing as inferiority or superiority in this matter. Man is not superior to woman, nor woman to man. The relation of the sexes is one of equality, not of better and worse, or of higher and lower. By this it is not intended to say that the sexes are the same. They are different, widely different from each other, and so different that each can do, in certain directions, what the other cannot; and in other directions, where both can do the same things, one sex, as a rule, can do them better than the other; and in still other matters they seem to be so nearly alike, that they can interchange labor without perceptible difference. All this is so well known, that it would be useless to refer to it,

were it not that much of the discussion of
the irrepressible woman-question, and many
of the efforts for bettering her education and
widening her sphere, seem to ignore any difference of the sexes; seem to treat her as if
she were identical with man, and to be trained
in precisely the same way; as if her organization, and consequently her function, were masculine, not feminine. There are those who
write and act as if their object were to assimi-
late woman as much as possible to man, by
dropping all that is distinctively feminine out
of her, and putting into her as large an
amount of masculineness as possible. These
persons tacitly admit the error just alluded to,
that woman is inferior to man, and strive to
get rid of the inferiority by making her a man.
There may be some subtle physiological basis
for such views — some strange quality of
brain; for some who hold and advocate
them are of those, who, having missed the
symmetry and organic balance that harmonious development yields, have drifted into
an hermaphroditic condition. One of this

class, who was glad to have escaped the
chains of matrimony, but knew the value and
lamented the loss of maternity, wished she
had been born a widow with two children.
These misconceptions arise from mistaking difference of organization and function for difference of position in the scale of being, which
is equivalent to saying that man is rated
higher in the divine order because he has more
muscle, and woman lower because she has
more fat. The loftiest ideal of humanity, re-
jecting all comparisons of inferiority and su
periority between the sexes, demands that each
shall be perfect in its kind, and not be hin-
dered in its best work. The lily is not inferior to the rose, nor the oak superior to the
clover : yet the glory of the lily is one, and
the glory of the oak is another ; and the use
of the oak is not the use of the clover. That
is poor horticulture which would train them
all alike.

When Col. Higginson asked, not long ago,
in one of his charming essays, that almost
persuade the reader, " Ought women to learn

the alphabet ? " and added, " Give woman, if
you dare, the alphabet, then summon her to
the career," his physiology was not equal
to his wit.   Women will learn the alphabet
at any rate; and man will be powerless to prevent them, should he undertake so ungracious
a task.   The real question is not, *Shall* women
learn the alphabet ? but *How* shall they learn
it ?   In this case, how is more important than
ought or shall.   The principle and duty are
not denied.   The method is not so plain.

The fact that women have often equalled
and sometimes excelled men in physical
labor, intellectual effort, and lofty heroism, is
sufficient proof that women have muscle,
mind, and soul, as well as men ; but it is no
proof that they have had, or should have, the
same kind of training ; nor is it any proof that
they are destined for the same career as men.
The presumption is, that if woman, subjected
to a masculine training, arranged for the
development of a masculine organization, can
equal man, she ought to excel him if educated
by a feminine training, arranged to develop a

feminine organization. Indeed, I have somewhere encountered an author who boldly affirms the superiority of women to all existences on this planet, because of the complexity of their organization. Without undertaking to indorse such an opinion, it may be affirmed, that an appropriate method of education for girls — one that should not ignore the mechanism of their bodies or blight any of their vital organs — would yield a better result than the world has yet seen.

Gail Hamilton's statement is true, that, " a girl can go to school, pursue all the studies which Dr. Todd enumerates, except *ad infinitum ;* know them, not as well as a chemist knows chemistry or a botanist botany, but as well as they are known by boys of her age and training, as well, indeed, as they are known by many college-taught men, enough, at least, to be a solace and a resource to her ; then graduate before she is eighteen, and come out of school as healthy, as fresh, as eager, as she went in." * But it is not true

---

* Woman's Wrongs, p. 59.

that she can do all this, and retain uninjured health and a future secure from neuralgia, uterine disease, hysteria, and other derangements of the nervous system, if she follows the same method that boys are trained in. Boys must study and work in a boy's way, and girls in a girl's way. They may study the same books, and attain an equal result, but should not follow the same method. Mary can master Virgil and Euclid as well as George ; but both will be dwarfed, — defrauded of their rightful attainment, — if both are confined to the same methods. It is said that Elena Cornaro, the accomplished professor of six languages, whose statue adorns and honors Padua, was educated like a boy. This means that she was initiated into, and mastered, the studies that were considered to be the peculiar dower of men. It does not mean that her life was a man's life, her way of study a man's way of study, or that, in acquiring six languages, she ignored her own organization. Women who choose to do so can master the humanities and the mathematics, encounter the labor of the law and the pulpit, endure the hardness of physic and the conflicts of politics ; but they must do it all in woman's way, not in man's way. In all their work they must respect their own organization, and remain women, not strive to be men, or they will ignominiously fail. For both sexes, there is no exception to the law, that their greatest power and largest attainment lie in the perfect development of their organization. " Woman," says a late writer, " must be regarded as woman, not as a nondescript animal, with greater or less capacity for assimilation to man." If we would give our girls a fair chance, and see them become and do their best by reaching after and attaining an ideal beauty and power, which shall be a crown of glory and a tower of strength to the republic, we must look after their complete development as women. Wherein they are men, they should be educated as men ; wherein they are women, they should be educated as women. The physiological motto is, Educate a man for manhood, a woman for womanhood, both for humanity. In this lies the hope of the race.

Perhaps it should be mentioned in this connection, that, throughout this paper, education
is not used in the limited and technical sense
of intellectual or mental training alone. By
saying there is a boy's way of study and a
girl's way of study, it is not asserted that the
intellectual process which masters Juvenal,
German, or chemistry, is different for the two
sexes. Education is here intended to include
what its etymology indicates, the drawing out
and development of every part of the system ;
and this necessarily includes the whole manner of life, physical and psychical, during the
educational period. "Education," says Worcester, "comprehends all that series of instruction and discipline which is intended to
enlighten the understanding, correct the tem-
per, and form the manners and habits, of
youth, and fit them for usefulness in their future stations." It has been and is the mis-
fortune of this country, and particularly of
New England, that education, stripped of this,
its proper signification, has popularly stood
for studying, without regard to the physical

training or no training that the schools afford. The cerebral processes by which the
acquisition of knowledge is made are the same
for each sex; but the mode of life which gives
the finest nurture to the brain, and so enables
those processes to yield their best result, is
not the same for each sex. The best educational training for a boy is not the best for a
girl, nor that for a girl best for a boy.

The delicate bloom, early but rapidly fad-
ing beauty, and singular pallor of American
girls and women have almost passed into a
proverb. The first observation of a European that lands upon our shores is, that our
women are a feeble race ; and, if he is a physiological observer, he is sure to add, They
will give birth to a feeble race, not of women
only, but of men as well. " I never saw
before so many pretty girls together," said
Lady Amberley to the writer, after a visit to
the public schools of Boston ; and then added,
" They all looked sick." Circumstances have
repeatedly carried me to Europe, where I am
always surprised by the red blood that fills

and colors the faces of ladies and peasant girls, reminding one of the canvas of Rubens and Murillo; and am always equally surprised on my return, by crowds of pale, bloodless female faces, that suggest consumption, scrofula, anemia, and neuralgia. To a large extent, our present system of educating girls is the cause of this palor and weakness. How our schools, through their methods of education, contribute to this unfortunate result, and how our colleges that have undertaken to educate girls like boys, that is, in the same way, have succeeded in intensifying the evils of the schools, will be pointed out in another place.

It has just been said that the educational methods of our schools and colleges for girls are, to a large extent, the cause of " the thousand ills " that beset American women. Let it be remembered that this is not asserting that such methods of education are the sole cause of female weaknesses, but only that they are one cause, and one of the most important causes of it. An immense loss of female power may be fairly charged to irrational cooking and indigestible diet. We live in the zone of perpetual pie and dough-nut; and our girls revel in those unassimilable abominations. Much also may be credited to artificial deformities strapped to the spine, or piled on the head, much to corsets and skirts, and as much to the omission of clothing where it is needed as to excess where the body does not require it ; but, after the amplest allowance for these as causes of weakness, there remains a large margin of disease unaccounted for. Those grievous maladies which torture a woman's earthly existence, called leucorrhœa, amenorrhœa, dysmenorrhœa, chronic and acute ovaritis, prolapsus uteri, hysteria, neuralgia, and the like, are indirectly affected by food, clothing, and exercise ; they are directly and largely affected by the causes that will be presently pointed out, and which arise from a neglect of the peculiarities of a woman's organization. The regimen of our schools fosters this neglect. The regimen of a college arranged for

boys, if imposed on girls, would foster it still
more.

The scope of this paper does not permit
the discussion of these other causes of female
weaknesses.   Its object is to call attention to
the errors of physical training that have crept
into, and twined themselves about, our ways
of educating girls, both in public and private
schools, and which now threaten to attain a
larger development, and inflict a consequently
greater injury, by their introduction into colleges and large seminaries of learning, that
have adopted, or are preparing to adopt, the
co-education of the sexes.   Even if there
were space to do so, it would not be necessary to discuss here the other causes alluded
to.   They are receiving the amplest attention
elsewhere.   The gifted authoress of " The
Gates Ajar " has blown her trumpet with no
uncertain sound, in explanation and advocacy
of a new-clothes philosophy, which her sisters will do well to heed rather than to ridi-
cule.   It would be a blessing to the race, if
some inspired prophet of clothes would ap-

pear, who should teach the coming woman
how, in pharmaceutical phrase, to fit, put on,
wear, and take off her dress, —

" Cito, Tuto, et Jucunde."

Corsets that embrace the waist with a tighter
and steadier grip than any lover's arm, and
skirts that weight the hips with heavier than
maternal burdens, have often caused grievous
maladies, and imposed a needless invalidism.
Yet, recognizing all this, it must not be forgotten that breeches do not make a man, nor
the want of them unmake a woman.

Let the statement be emphasized and re-
iterated until it is heeded, that woman's neglect of her own organization, though not the
sole explanation and cause of her many weaknesses, more than any single cause, adds to
their number, and intensifies their power. It
limits and lowers her action very much, as
man is limited and degraded by dissipation.
The saddest part of it all is, that this neglect
of herself in girlhood, when her organization
is ductile and impressible, breeds the germs

of diseases that in later life yield torturing
or fatal maladies.   Every physician's note-
book affords copious illustrations of these
statements.   The number of them which the
writer has seen prompted this imperfect
essay upon a subject in which the public has
a most vital interest, and with regard to
which it acts with the courage of ignorance.

Two considerations deserve to be mentioned in this connection.   One is, that no
organ or function in plant, animal, or human
kind, can be properly regarded as a disability
or source of weakness.   Through ignorance or
misdirection, it may limit or enfeeble the animal or being that misguides it; but, rightly
guided and developed, it is either in itself a
source of power and grace to its parent stock,
or a necessary stage in the development of
larger grace and power.   The female organization is no exception to this law; nor are the
particular set of organs and their functions
with which this essay has to deal an exception
to it.   The periodical movements which characterize and influence woman's structure for

more than half her terrestrial life, and which, in their ebb and flow, sway every fibre and thrill every nerve of her body a dozen times a year, and the occasional pregnancies which test her material resources, and cradle the race, are, or are evidently intended to be, fountains of power, not hinderances, to her. They are not infrequently spoken of by women themselves with half-smothered anathemas; often endured only as a necessary evil and sign of inferiority; and commonly ignored, till some steadily-advancing malady whips the recalcitrant sufferer into acknowledgment of their power, and respect for their function. All this is a sad mistake. It is a foolish and criminal delicacy that has persuaded woman to be so ashamed of the temple God built for her as to neglect one of its most important services. On account of this neglect, each succeeding generation, obedient to the law of hereditary transmission, has become feebler than its predecessor. Our great-grandmothers are pointed at as types of female physical excellence; their great - grand - daughters as illustrations of female physical degeneracy. There is con solation, however, in the hope, based on substantial physiological data, that our great-grand-daughters may recapture their ancestors' bloom and force. " Three generations of wholesome life," says Mr. Greg, " might suffice to eliminate the ancestral poison, for the *vis medicatrix naturæ* has wonderful efficacy when allowed free play; and perhaps the time may come when the worst cases shall deem it a plain duty to curse no future generations with the *damnosa hereditas*, which has caused such bitter wretchedness to themselves." *

The second consideration is the acknowledged influence of beauty. " When one sees a god-like countenance," said Socrates to Phædrus, " or some bodily form that represents beauty, he reverences it as a god, and would sacrifice to it." From the days of Plato till now, all have felt the power of woman's beauty, and been more than willing

* Enigmas of Life, p. 34.

to sacrifice to it. The proper, not exclusive
search for it is a legitimate inspiration. The
way for a girl to obtain her portion of this
radiant halo is by the symmetrical development of every part of her organization,
muscle, ovary, stomach and nerve, and by a
physiological management of every function
that correlates every organ; not by neglecting or trying to stifle or abort any of the
vital and integral parts of her structure, and
supplying the deficiency by invoking the aid
of the milliner's stuffing, the colorist's pencil,
the druggist's compounds, the doctor's pelvic
supporter, and the surgeon's spinal brace.

When travelling in the East, some years
ago, it was my fortune to be summoned as a
physician into a harem. With curious and
not unwilling step I obeyed the summons.
While examining the patient, nearly a dozen
Syrian girls — a grave Turk's wifely crowd,
his matrimonial bouquet and armful of con-
nubial bliss — pressed around the divan with
eyes and ears intent to see and hear a Western
Hakim's medical examination. As I looked

upon their well-developed forms, their brown skins, rich with the blood and sun of the East, and their unintelligent, sensuous faces, I thought that if it were possible to marry the Oriental care of woman's organization to the Western liberty and culture of her brain, there would be a new birth and loftier type of womanly grace and force.

PART II.

" She girdeth her loins with strength." — Solomon.

BEFORE describing the special forms of ill that exist among our American, certainly among our New-England girls and women, and that are often caused and fostered by our methods of education and social customs, it is important to refer in considerable detail to a few physiological matters. Physiology serves to disclose the cause, and explain the *modus operandi*, of these ills, and offers the only rational clew to their prevention and relief. The order in which the physiological data are presented that bear upon this discussion is not essential; their relation to the subject matter of it will be obvious as we proceed.

31

The sacred number, three, dominates the human frame. There is a trinity in our anatomy. Three systems, to which all the organs are directly or indirectly subsidiary, divide and control the body. First, there is the nutritive system, composed of stomach, intestines, liver, pancreas, glands, and vessels, by which food is elaborated, effete matter removed, the blood manufactured, and the whole organization nourished. This is the commissariat. Secondly, there is the nervous system, which co-ordinates all the organs and functions; which enables man to entertain relations with the world around him, and with his fellows; and through which intellectual power is manifested, and human thought and reason made possible. Thirdly, there is the reproductive system, by which the race is continued, and its grasp on the earth assured. The first two of these systems are alike in each sex. They are so alike, that they require a similar training in each, and yield in each a similar result. The machinery of them is the same. No scalpel has disclosed any difference between a man's and a woman's liver. No microscope has revealed any structure, fibre, or cell, in the brain of man or woman, that is not common to both. No analysis or dynamemeter has discovered or measured any chemical action or nerve-force that stamps either of these systems as male or female. From these anatomical and physiological data alone, the inference is legitimate, that intellectual power, the correlation and measure of cerebral structure and metamorphosis, is capable of equal development in both sexes. With regard to the reproductive system, the case is altogether different. Woman, in the interest of the race, is dowered with a set of organs peculiar to herself, whose complexity, delicacy, sympathies, and force are among the marvels of creation. If properly nurtured and cared for, they are a source of strength and power to her. If neglected and mismanaged, they retaliate upon their possessor with weakness and disease, as well of the mind as of the body. God was not in error, when, after Eve's creation, he looked upon his work, and pro-

nounced it good.   Let Eve take a wise care
of the temple God made for her, and Adam
of the one made for him, and both will enter
upon a career whose glory and beauty no
seer has foretold or poet sung.

Ever since the time of Hippocrates, woman
has been physiologically described as enjoying,
and has always recognized herself as enjoying,
or at least as possessing, a tri-partite life. The
first period extends from birth to about the
age of twelve or fifteen years; the second,
from the end of the first period to about the
age of forty-five ; and the third, from the last
boundary to the final passage into the unknown.   The few years that are necessary
for the voyage from the first to the second
period, and those from the second to the
third, are justly called critical ones. Mothers
are, or should be, wisely anxious about the
first passage for their daughters, and women
are often unduly apprehensive about the
second passage for themselves. All this is
obvious and known ; and yet, in our educational arrangements, little heed is paid to

the fact, that the first of these critical
voyages is made during a girl's educational
life, and extends over a very considerable
portion of it.

This brief statement only hints at the vital
physiological truths it contains: it does not
disclose them. Let us look at some of them
a moment. Remember, that we are now concerned only with the first of these passages,
that from a girl's childhood to her maturity.
In childhood, boys and girls are very nearly
alike. If they are natural, they talk and
romp, chase butterflies and climb fences, love
and hate, with an innocent *abandon* that is
ignorant of sex. Yet even then the difference is apparent to the observing. Inspired
by the divine instinct of motherhood, the girl
that can only creep to her mother's knees will
caress a doll, that her tottling brother looks
coldly upon. The infant Achilles breaks the
thin disguise of his gown and sleeves by dropping the distaff, and grasping the sword. As
maturity approaches, the sexes diverge. An
unmistakable difference marks the form and

features of each, and reveals the demand for a special training. This divergence, however, is limited in its sweep and its duration. The difference exists for a definite purpose, and goes only to a definite extent. The curves of separation swell out as childhood recedes, like an ellipse, and, as old age draws on, approach, till they unite like an ellipse again. In old age, the second childhood, the difference of sex becomes of as little note as it was during the first. At that period, the picture of the

> " Lean and slippered pantaloon,
> With spectacles on nose, and pouch on side,
>
> .   .   .   .
>
> Sans teeth, sans eyes, sans taste, sans every thing,"

is faithful to either sex. Not as man or woman, but as a sexless being, does advanced age enter and pass the portals of what is called death.

During the first of these critical periods, when the divergence of the sexes becomes obvious to the most careless observer, the complicated apparatus peculiar to the female enters upon a condition of functional activity.

"The ovaries, which constitute," says Dr. Dalton, "the 'essential parts' * of this apparatus, and certain accessory organs, are now rapidly developed." Previously they were inactive. During infancy and childhood all of them existed, or rather all the germs of them existed; but they were incapable of function. At this period they take on a process of rapid growth and development. Coincident with this process, indicating it, and essential to it, are the periodical phenomena which characterize woman's physique till she attains the third division of her tripartite life. The growth of this peculiar and marvellous apparatus, in the perfect development of which humanity has so large an interest, occurs during the few years of a girl's educational life. No such extraordinary task, calling for such rapid expenditure of force, building up such a delicate and extensive mechanism within the organism, — a house within a house, an engine within an engine, — is imposed upon the male

* Human Physiology, p. 546.

physique at the same epoch.*   The organization of the male grows steadily, gradually,
and equally, from birth to maturity.   The
importance of having our methods of female
education recognize this peculiar demand for
growth, and of so adjusting themselves to
it, as to allow a sufficient opportunity for
the healthy development of the ovaries and
their accessory organs, and for the estab-
lishment of their periodical functions, can
not be overestimated.   Moreover, unless the
work is accomplished at that period, unless
the reproductive mechanism is built and
put in good working order at that time,
it is never perfectly accomplished afterwards.
" It is not enough," says Dr. Charles

* As might be expected, the mortality of girls is greater at
this period than that of boys, an additional reason for im-
posing less labor on the former at that time.   According to
the authority of M.M. Quetelet and Smits, the mortality of
the two sexes is equal in childhood, or that of the male is
greatest; but that of the female rises between the ages of
fourteen and sixteen to 1.28 to one male death.   For the next
four years, it falls again to 1.05 females to one male death.
— *Sur la Reproduction et la Mortalité de l'Homme. 8vo. Brux-
elles.*

West, the accomplished London physician, and lecturer on diseases of women, "it is not enough to take precautions till menstruation has for the first time occurred : the period for its return should, even in the healthiest girl, be watched for, and all previous precautions should be once more repeated ; and this should be done again and again, until at length the *habit* of regular, healthy menstruation is established. If this be not accomplished during the first few years of womanhood, it will, in all probability, never be attained." * There have been instances, and I have seen such, of females in whom the special mechanism we are speaking of remained germinal,—undeveloped. It seemed to have been aborted. They graduated from school or college excellent scholars, but with undeveloped ovaries. Later they married, and were sterile. †

---

* Lectures on Diseases of Women. Am. ed., p. 48.

† "Much less uncommon than the absence of either ovary is the persistence of both through the whole or greater part of life in the condition which they present in infancy and early childhood, with scarcely a trace of graafian vesicles in

The system never does two things well at
the same time.   The muscles and the brain
cannot *functionate* in their best way at the
same moment.   One cannot meditate a poem
and drive a saw simultaneously, without dividing his force.   He may poetize fairly, and
saw poorly ; or he may saw fairly, and poetize
poorly ; or he may both saw and poetize in-
differently.   Brain-work and stomach-work
interfere with each other if attempted together.   The digestion of a dinner calls force
to the stomach, and temporarily slows the
brain.   The experiment of trying to digest a
hearty supper, and to sleep during the process,
has sometimes cost the careless experimenter
his life.   The physiological principle of doing
only one thing at a time, if you would do it
well, holds as truly of the growth of the organization as it does of the performance of

their tissue.   This want of development of the ovaries is
generally, though not invariably, associated with want of
development of the uterus and other sexual organs ; and I
need not say that women in whom it exists are sterile." —
Lectures on the Diseases of Women, by Charles West, M.D
Am. ed., p. 37.

any of its special functions. If excessive labor, either mental or physical, is imposed upon children, male or female, their development will be in some way checked. If the schoolmaster overworks the brains of his pupils, he diverts force to the brain that is needed elsewhere. He spends in the study of geography and arithmetic, of Latin, Greek and chemistry, in the brain-work of the school room, force that should have been spent in the manufacture of blood, muscle, and nerve, that is, in growth. The results are monstrous brains and puny bodies ; abnormally active cerebration, and abnormally weak digestion ; flowing thought and constipated bowels ; lofty aspirations and neuralgic sensations ;

" A youth of study and an old age of *nerves.*"

Nature has reserved the catamenial week for the process of ovulation, and for the development and perfection of the reproductive system. Previously to the age of eighteen or twenty, opportunity must be periodically allowed for the accomplishment of this task.

Both muscular and brain labor must be remitted enough to yield sufficient force for the
work.   If the reproductive machinery is not
manufactured then, it will not be later.
If it is imperfectly made then, it can only be
patched up, not made perfect, afterwards. To
be well made, it must be carefully managed.
Force must be allowed to flow thither in an
ample stream, and not diverted to the brain by
the school, or to the arms by the factory, or to
the feet by dancing. " Every physician,"
says a recent writer, " can point to students
whose splendid cerebral development has been
paid for by emaciated limbs, enfeebled digestion, and disordered lungs.   Every biography
of the intellectual great records the dangers
they have encountered, often those to which
they have succumbed, in overstepping the
ordinary bounds of human capacity ; and
while beckoning onward to the glories of
their almost preternatural achievements, re-
gister, by way of warning, the fearful penalty
of disease, suffering, and bodily infirmity,
which Nature exacts as the price for this par-

tial and inharmonious grandeur. It cannot be otherwise. The brain cannot take more than its share without injury to other organs. It cannot *do* more than its share without depriving other organs of that exercise and nourishment which are essential to their health and vigor. It is in the power of the individual to throw, as it were, the whole vigor of the constitution into any one part, and, by giving to this part exclusive or excessive attention, to develop it at the expense, and to the neglect, of the others." *

In the system of lichens, Nylander reckons all organs of equal value.† No one of them can be neglected without evil to the whole organization. From lichens to men and women there is no exception to the law, that, if one member suffers, all the members suffer. What is true of the neglect of a single organ, is true in a geometrical ratio of the neglect of a system of organs. If the nutritive system is wrong, the evil of poor nourishment and

---

* Enigmas of Life, pp. 165–8.

† Tuckerman's Genera Lichenum. Introduction, p. v

bad assimilation infects the whole economy. Brain and thought are enfeebled, because the stomach and liver are in error. If the nervous system is abnormally developed, every organ feels the *twist* in the nerves. The balance and co-ordination of movement and function are destroyed, and the ill percolates into an unhappy posterity. If the reproductive system is aborted, there may be no future generations to pay the penalty of the abortion, but what is left of the organism suffers sadly. When this sort of arrest of development occurs in a man, it takes the element of masculineness out of him, and replaces it with adipose effeminacy. When it occurs in a woman, it not only substitutes in her case a wiry and perhaps thin bearded masculineness for distinctive feminine traits and power, making her an epicene, but it entails a variety of prolonged weaknesses, that dwarf her rightful power in almost every direction. The persistent neglect and ignoring by women, and especially by girls, ignorantly more than wilfully, of that part of

their organization which they hold in trust
for the future of the race, has been fearfully
punished here in America, where, of all the
world, they are least trammelled and should
be the best, by all sorts of female trou-
bles. " Nature," says Lord Bacon, " is
often hidden, sometimes overcome, seldom
extinguished." In the education of our
girls, the attempt to hide or overcome nature
by training them as boys has almost extinguished them as girls. Let the fact be accepted, that there is nothing to be ashamed
of in a woman's organization, and let her
whole education and life be guided by the
divine requirements of her system.

The blood, which is our life, is a complex
fluid. It contains the materials out of which
the tissues are made, and also the *débris*
which results from the destruction of the
same tissues, — the worn-out cells of brain
and muscle, — the cast-off clothes of emotion,
thought, and power. It is a common carrier,
conveying unceasingly to every gland and
tissue, to every nerve and organ, the fibrin

and albumen which repair their constant
waste, thus supplying their daily bread; and
as unceasingly conveying away from every
gland and tissue, from every nerve and organ,
the oxidized refuse, which are both the result
and measure of their work. Like the water
flowing through the canals of Venice, that
carries health and wealth to the portals of
every house, and filth and disease from every
doorway, the blood flowing through the
canals of the organization carries nutriment
to all the tissues, and refuse from them. Its
current sweeps nourishment in, and waste
out. The former, it yields to the body for
assimilation; the latter, it deposits with the
organs of elimination for rejection. In order
to have good blood, then, two things are essential: first, a regular and sufficient supply
of nutriment, and, secondly, an equally regular and sufficient removal of waste. Insufficient nourishment starves the blood;
insufficient elimination poisons it. A wise
housekeeper will look as carefully after the
condition of his drains as after the quality

The principal organs of elimination, common to both sexes, are the bowels, kidneys, lungs, and skin. A neglect of their functions is punished in each alike. To woman is intrusted the exclusive management of another process of elimination, viz., the catamenial function. This, using the blood for its channel of operation, performs, like the blood, double duty. It is necessary to ovulation, and to the integrity of every part of the reproductive apparatus; it also serves as a means of elimination for the blood itself. A careless management of this function, at any period of life during its existence, is apt to be followed by consequences that may be serious; but a neglect of it during the epoch of development, that is, from the age of fourteen to eighteen or twenty, not only produces great evil at the time of the neglect, but leaves a large legacy of evil to the future. The system is then peculiarly susceptible; and disturbances of the delicate mechanism we are considering, induced during the catamenial weeks of that critical age by constrained positions, muscular effort, brain

work, and all forms of mental and physical
excitement, germinate a host of ills. Sometimes these causes, which pervade more or less
the methods of instruction in our public and
private schools, which our social customs ignore, and to which operatives of all sorts pay
little heed, produce an excessive performance
of the catamenial function ; and this is equivalent to a periodical hemorrhage. Sometimes
they produce an insufficient performance of
it ; and this, by closing an avenue of elimination, poisons the blood, and depraves the organization. The host of ills thus induced are
known to physicians and to the sufferers as
amenorrhœa, menorrhagia, dysmenorrhœa,
hysteria, anemia, chorea, and the like. Some
of these fasten themselves on their victim for
a lifetime, and some are shaken off. Now and
then they lead to an abortion of the function,
and consequent sterility. Fortunate is the
girls' school or college that does not furnish
abundant examples of these sad cases. The
more completely any such school or college
succeeds, while adopting every detail and

method of a boy's school, in ignoring and neglecting the physiological conditions of sexual development, the larger will be the number of these pathological cases among its graduates. Clinical illustrations of these statements will be given in another place.

The mysterious process which physiologists call metamorphosis of tissue, or intestitial change, deserves attention in connection with our subject. It interests both sexes alike. Unless it goes on normally, neither boys, girls, men, nor women, can have bodies or brains worth talking about. It is a process, without which not a step can be taken, or muscle moved, or food digested, or nutriment assimilated, or any function, physical or mental, performed. By its aid, growth and development are carried on. Youth, maturity, and old age result from changes in its character. It is alike the support and the guide of health convalescence, and disease. It is the means by which, in the human system, force is developed, and growth and decay rendered possible. The process, in itself, is one of the simplest. It is merely the replacing of one microscopic cell by another; and yet upon this simple process hang the issues of life and death, of thought and power.

Carpenter, in his physiology, reports the discovery, which we owe to German investigation, "that the whole structure originates in a single cell; that this cell gives birth to others, analogous to itself, and these again to many future generations; and that all the varied tissues of the animal body are developed from cells."* A more recent writer adds, "In the higher animals and plants, we are presented with structures which may be regarded as essentially aggregates of cells; and there is now a physiological division of labor, some of the cells being concerned with the nutriment of the organism, whilst others are set apart, and dedicated to the function of reproduction. Every cell in such an aggregate leads a life, which, in a certain limited sense, may be said to be independent; and each discharges its own function in the

---

* Carpenter's Human Physiology, p. 455.

general economy. Each cell has a period of development, growth, and active life, and each ultimately perishes; the life of the organism not only not depending upon the life of its elemental factors, but actually being kept up by their constant destruction and as constant renewal." * Growth, health, and disease are cellular manifestations. With every act of life, the movement of a finger, the pulsation of a heart, the uttering of a word, the coining of a thought, the thrill of an emotion, there is the destruction of a certain number of cells. Their destruction evolves or sets free the force that we recognize as movement, speech, thought, and emotion. The number of cells destroyed depends upon the intensity and duration of the effort that correlates their destruction. When a blacksmith wields a hammer for an hour, he uses up the number of cells necessary to yield that amount of muscular force. When a girl studies Latin for an hour, she uses up the number of brain-cells necessary

---

* Nicholson, Study of Biology, p. 79.

to yield that amount of intellectual force.
As fast as one cell is destroyed, another is
generated. The death of one is followed
instantly by the birth of its successor. This
continual process of cellular death and birth,
the income and outgo of cells, that follow
each other like the waves of the sea, each
different yet each the same, is metamorphosis
of tissue. This is life. It corresponds very
nearly to Bichat's definition that, " life is
organization in action." The finer sense of
Shakspeare dictated a truer definition than
the science of the French physiologist, —

> " What's yet in this
> That bears the name of life ?   Yet in this life
> Lie hid more thousand deaths."
>
> *Measure for Measure*, Act iii. Scene 1.

No physical or psychical act is possible
without this change. It is a process of continual waste and repair. Subject to its inevitable power, the organization is continually
wasting away and continually being repaired.

The old notion that our bodies are changed

every seven years, science has long since exploded. "The matter," said Mr. John Goodsir, "of the organized frame to its minutest parts is in a continual flux." Our bodies are never the same for any two successive days. The feet that Mary shall dance with next Christmas Eve will not be the same feet that bore her triumphantly through the previous Christmas holidays. The brain that she learns German with today does not contain a cell in its convolutions that was spent in studying French one year ago. Whether her present feet can dance better or worse than those of a year ago, and whether her present brain can *do* more or less German and French than the one of the year before, depends upon how she has used her feet and brain during the intervening time, that is, upon the metamorphosis of her tissue.

From birth to adult age, the cells of muscle, organ, and brain that are spent in the activities of life, such as digesting, growing, studying, playing, working, and the like, are replaced by others of better quality and larger number. At least, such is the case where metamorphosis is permitted to go on normally. The result is growth and development. This growing period or formative epoch extends from birth to the age of twenty or twenty-five years. Its duration is shorter for a girl than for a boy. She ripens quicker than he. In the four years from fourteen to eighteen, she accomplishes an amount of physiological cell change and growth which Nature does not require of a boy in less than twice that number of years. It is obvious, that to secure the best kind of growth during this period, and the best development at the end of it, the waste of tissue produced by study, work, and fashion must not be so great that repair will only equal it. It is equally obvious that a girl upon whom Nature, for a limited period and for a definite purpose, imposes so great a physiological task, will not have as much power left for the tasks of the school, as the boy of whom Nature requires less at the corresponding epoch. A margin must be allowed for growth. The repair must be greater and better than the waste.

During middle age, life's active period, there is an equilibrium between the body's waste and repair: one equals the other. The machine, when properly managed, then holds its own. A French physiologist fixes the close of this period for the ideal man of the future at eighty, when, he says, old age begins. Few have such inherited power, and live with such physiological wisdom, as to keep their machine in good repair, — in good working-order, — to that late period. From the age of twenty-five or thirty, however, to that of sixty or sixty-five, this equilibrium occurs. Repair then equals waste; reconstruction equals destruction. The female organization, like the male, is now developed: its tissues are consolidated; its functions are established. With decent care, it can perform an immense amount of physical and mental labor. It is now capable of its best work. But, in order to do its best, it must

obey the law of periodicity; just as the
male organization, to do its best, must obey
the law of sustained effort.

When old age begins, whether, normally,
at seventy or eighty, or, prematurely, at fifty
or thirty, repair does not equal waste, and
degeneration of tissue results. More cells
are destroyed by wear and tear than are
made up from nutriment. The friction of
the machine rubs the stuff of life away faster
than it can be replaced. The muscles stiffen,
the hair turns white, the joints crack, the
arteries ossify, the nerve-centres harden or
soften: all sorts of degeneration creep on
till death appears, — *Mors janua vitæ.* There
the curves unite, and men and women are
alike again.

Sleep, whose inventor received the bene-
diction of Sancho Panza, and whose power
Dryden apostrophized, —

> " Of all the powers the best :
> Oh ! peace of mind, repairer of decay,
> Whose balm renews the limbs to labor of the day," —

is a most important physiological factor.

Our schools are as apt in frightening it away as our churches are in inviting it. Sleep is the opportunity for repair. During its hours of quiet rest, when muscular and nervous effort are stilled, millions of microscopic cells are busy in the penetralia of the organism, like coral insects in the depths of the sea, repairing the waste which the day's study and work have caused. Dr. B. W. Richardson of London, one of the most ingenious and accomplished physiologists of the present day, describes the labor of sleep in the following language: "During this period of natural sleep, the most important changes of nutrition are in progress: the body is renovating, and, if young, is actually growing. If the body be properly covered, the animal heat is being conserved, and laid up for expenditure during the waking hours that are to follow; the respiration is reduced, the inspirations being lessened in the proportion of six to seven, as compared with the number made when the body is awake; the action of the heart is reduced; the voluntary muscles, relieved of all fatigue, and with the extensors more relaxed than the flexors, are undergoing repair of structure, and recruiting their excitability ; and the voluntary nervous system, dead for the time to the external vibration, or, as the older men called it, ' stimulus' from without, is also undergoing rest and repair, so that, when it comes again into work, it may receive better the impressions it may have to gather up, and influence more effectively the muscles it may be called upon to animate, direct, control." *

An American observer and physiologist, Dr. William A. Hammond, confirms the views of his English colleague. He tells us that " the state of general repose which accompanies sleep is of especial value to the organism, in allowing the nutrition of the nervous tissue to go on at a greater rate than its destructive metamorphosis." In another place he adds, " For the brain, there is no rest except during sleep." And, again, he says, " The more active the mind, the

---

* Popular Science Monthly, August, 1872, p. 411.

greater the necessity for sleep ; just as with a steamer, the greater the number of revolutions its engine makes, the more imperative is the demand for fuel." * These statements justify and explain the instinctive demand for sleep. They also show why it is that infants require more sleep than children, and children than middle-age folk, and middle-age folk than old people. Infants must have sleep for repair and rapid growth ; children, for repair and moderate growth ; middle-age folk, for repair without growth ; and old people, only for the minimum of repair. Girls, between the ages of fourteen and eighteen, must have sleep, not only for repair and growth, like boys, but for the additional task of constructing, or, more properly speaking, of developing and perfecting then, a reproductive system, — the engine within an engine. The bearing of this physiological fact upon education is obvious. Work of the school is work of the brain. Work of the brain eats the brain away. Sleep is the chance

---

* Sleep and its Derangements, pp. 9, 10, 13.

and laboratory of repair. If a child's brain-
work and sleep are normally proportioned to
each other, each night will more than make
good each day's loss. Clear heads will greet
each welcome morn. But if the reverse
occurs, the night will not repair the day;
and aching heads will signalize the advance
of neuralgia, tubercle, and disease. So Nature
punishes disobedience.

It is apparent, from these physiological
considerations, that, in order to give girls a
fair chance in education, four conditions at
least must be observed: first, a sufficient
supply of appropriate nutriment; secondly, a
normal management of the catamenial functions, including the building of the reproductive apparatus; thirdly, mental and physical
work so apportioned, that repair shall exceed
waste, and a margin be left for general and
sexual development; and fourthly, sufficient
sleep. Evidence of the results brought about
by a disregard of these conditions will next
be given.

PART III.

CHIEFLY CLINICAL.

"Et l'on nous persuadera difficilement que lorsque les hommes ont tant de peine à être hommes, les femmes puissent, tout en restant femmes, devenir hommes aussi, mettant ainsi la main sur les deux rôles, exerçant la double mission, résumant le double caractère de l'humanité ! Nous perdrons la femme, et nous n'aurons pas l'homme. Voila ce qui nous arrivera. On nous donnera ce quelque chose de monstreux, cet être répugnant, qui déjà parait à notre horizon."
— LE COMTE A. DE GASPARIN.

"Facts given in evidence are premises from which a conclusion is to be drawn. The first step in the exercise of this duty is to acquire a belief of the truth of the facts." — RAM, on *Facts*.

CLINICAL observation confirms the teachings of physiology. The sick chamber, not the schoolroom ; the physician's private consultation, not the committee's public examination ; the hospital, not the college, the

workshop, or the parlor, — disclose the sad
results which modern social customs, modern
education, and modern ways of labor, have
entailed on women. Examples of them may
be found in every walk of life. On the lux-
urious couches of Beacon Street; in the pal-
aces of Fifth Avenue; among the classes of
our private, common, and normal schools;
among the female graduates of our colleges;
behind the counters of Washington Street
and Broadway; in our factories, workshops,
and homes, — may be found numberless pale,
weak, neuralgic, dyspeptic, hysterical, men-
orrhœic, dysmenorrhœic girls and women,
that are living illustrations of the truth of
this brief monograph. It is not asserted here
that improper methods of study, and a disregard
of the reproductive apparatus and its functions, during the educational life of girls, are
the sole causes of female diseases; neither is
it asserted that all the female graduates of
our schools and colleges are pathological
specimens. But it is asserted that the number of these graduates who have been per-

manently disabled to a greater or less degree
by these causes is so great, as to excite the
gravest alarm, and to demand the serious
attention of the community. If these causes
should continue for the next half-century,
and increase in the same ratio as they have
for the last fifty years, it requires no prophet
to foretell that the wives who are to be
mothers in our republic must be drawn from
trans-atlantic homes. The sons of the New
World will have to re-act, on a magnificent
scale, the old story of unwived Rome and the
Sabines.

We have previously seen that the blood is
the life, and that the loss of it is the loss of
so much life. Deluded by strange theories,
and groping in physiological darkness, our
fathers' physicians were too often Sangrados.
Nourishing food, pure air, and hæmatized
blood were stigmatized as the friends of disease and the enemies of convalescence. Oxygen was shut out from and carbonic acid
shut into the chambers of phthisis and fever;
and veins were opened, that the currents of

blood and disease might flow out together. Happily, those days of ignorance, which God winked at, and which the race survived, have passed by. Air and food and blood are recognized as Nature's restoratives. No physician would dare, nowadays, to bleed either man or woman once a month, year in and year out, for a quarter of a century continuously. But girls often have the courage, or the ignorance, to do this to themselves. And the worst of it is, that the organization of our schools and workshops, and the demands of social life and polite society, encourage them in this slow suicide. It has already been stated that the excretory organs, by constantly eliminating from the system its effete and used material, the measure and source of its force, keep the machine in clean, healthy, and working order, and that the reproductive apparatus of woman uses the blood as one of its agents of elimination. Kept within natural limits, this elimination is a source of strength, a perpetual fountain of health, a constant renewal of life. Beyond

these limits it is a hemorrhage, that, by drain-
ing away the life, becomes a source of weakness and a perpetual fountain of disease.

The following case illustrates one of the
ways in which our present school methods of
teaching girls generate a menorrhagia and
its consequent evils. Miss A——, a healthy,
bright, intelligent girl, entered a female
school, an institution that is commonly but
oddly called a *seminary* for girls, in the State
of New York, at the age of fifteen. She was
then sufficiently-well developed, and had a
good color ; all the functions appeared to act
normally, and the catamenia were fairly established. She was ambitious as well as capable, and aimed to be among the first in the
school. Her temperament was what physiologists call nervous, — an expression that
does not denote a fidgety make, but refers
to a relative activity of the nervous system.
She was always anxious about her recitations.
No matter how carefully she prepared for
them, she was ever fearful lest she should
trip a little, and appear to less advantage

5

than she hoped. She went to school regularly every week, and every day of the school year, just as boys do. She paid no more attention to the periodical tides of her organization than her companions; and that was none at all. She recited standing at all times, or at least whenever a standing recitation was the order of the hour. She soon found, and this history is taken from her own lips, that for a few days during every fourth week, the effort of reciting produced an extraordinary physical result. The attendant anxiety and excitement relaxed the sluices of the system that were already physiologically open, and determined a hemorrhage as the concomitant of a recitation. Subjected to the inflexible rules of the school, unwilling to seek advice from any one, almost ashamed of her own physique, she ingeniously protected herself against exposure, and went on intellectually leading her companions, and physically defying nature. At the end of a year, she went home with a gratifying report from her teachers, and pale cheeks and a variety of aches. Her parents were pleased, and perhaps a little anxious. She is a good scholar, said her father; somewhat over-worked possibly; and so he gave her a trip among the mountains, and a week or two at the seashore. After her vacation she re-turned to school, and repeated the previous year's experience, — constant, sustained work, recitation and study for all days alike, a hem-orrhage once a month that would make the stroke oar of the University crew falter, and a brilliant scholar. Before the expiration of the second year, Nature began to assert her authority. The paleness of Miss A's com-plexion increased. An unaccountable and uncontrollable twitching of a rhythmical sort got into the muscles of her face, and made her hands go and feet jump. She was sent home, and her physician called, who at once diagnosticated chorea (St. Vitus' dance), and said she had studied too hard, and wisely prescribed no study and a long vaca-tion. Her parents took her to Europe. A year of the sea and the Alps, of England

and the Continent, the Rhine and Italy, worked like a charm. The sluiceways were controlled, the blood saved, and color and health returned. She came back seemingly well, and at the age of eighteen went to her old school once more. During all this time not a word had been said to her by her parents, her physician, or her teachers, about any periodical care of herself; and the rules of the school did not acknowledge the cata-menia. The labor and regimen of the school soon brought on the old menorrhagic trouble in the old way, with the addition of occasional faintings to emphasize Nature's warnings. She persisted in getting her education, however, and graduated at nineteen, the first scholar, and an invalid. Again her parents were gratified and anxious. She is overworked, said they, and wondered why girls break down so. To insure her recovery, a second and longer travel was undertaken. Egypt and Asia were added to Europe, and nearly two years were allotted to the cure. With change of air and scene her health im-

proved, but not so rapidly as with the previous journey. She returned to America
better than she went away, and married at
the age of twenty-two. Soon after that time
she consulted the writer on account of prolonged dyspepsia, neuralgia, and dysmenorrhœa, which had replaced menorrhagia. Then
I learned the long history of her education,
and of her efforts to study just as boys do.
Her attention had never been called before to
the danger she had incurred while at school.
She is now what is called getting better,
but has the delicacy and weaknesses of
American women, and, so far, is without
children.

It is not difficult, in this case, either to discern the cause of the trouble, or to trace its
influence, through the varying phases of
disease, from Miss A——'s school-days, to
her matronly life. She was well, and would
have been called robust, up to her first critical
period. She then had two tasks imposed
upon her at once, both of which required for
their perfect accomplishment a few years of

time and a large share of vital force : one
was the education of the brain, the other of
the reproductive system.   The schoolmaster
superintended the first, and Nature the
second.   The school, with puritanic inflexi-
bility, demanded every day of the month;
Nature, kinder than the school, demanded
less than a fourth of the time, — a seventh
or an eighth of it would have probably
answered.   The schoolmaster might have
yielded somewhat, but would not; Nature
could not.   The pupil, therefore, was compelled to undertake both tasks at the same
time.   Ambitious, earnest, and conscientious,
she obeyed the visible power and authority
of the school, and disobeyed, or rather ignorantly sought to evade, the invisible power
and authority of her organization.   She put
her will into the education of her brain, and
withdrew it from elsewhere.   The system
does not do two things well at the same time.
One or the other suffers from neglect, when
the attempt is made.   Miss A—— made her
brain and muscles work actively, and diverted

blood and force to them when her organization demanded active work, with blood and
force for evolution in another region. At
first the schoolmaster seemed to be successful. He not only made his pupil's brain
manipulate Latin, chemistry, philosophy,
geography, grammar, arithmetic, music,
French, German, and the whole extraordinary catalogue of an American young lady's
school curriculum, with acrobatic skill; but
he made her do this irrespective of the periodical tides of her organism, and made her
perform her intellectual and muscular calis-
thenics, obliging her to stand, walk, and
recite, at the seasons of highest tide. For a
while she got on nicely. Presently, however, the strength of the loins, that even
Solomon put in as a part of his ideal woman,
changed to weakness. Periodical hemorrhages were the first warning of this. As
soon as loss of blood occurred regularly and
largely, the way to imperfect development
and invalidism was open, and the progress
easy and rapid. The nerves and their centres

lacked nourishment. There was more waste than repair, — no margin for growth. St. Vitus' dance was a warning not to be neglected, and the schoolmaster resigned to the doctor. A long vacation enabled the system to retrace its steps, and recover force for evolution. Then the school resumed its sway, and physiological laws were again defied. Fortunately graduation soon occurred, and unintermitted, sustained labor was no longer enforced. The menorrhagia ceased, but persistent dysmenorrhea now indicates the neuralgic friction of an imperfectly developed reproductive apparatus. Doubtless the evil of her education will infect her whole life.

The next case is drawn from different social surroundings. Early associations and natural aptitude inclined Miss B—— to the stage ; and the need of bread and butter sent her upon it as a child, at what age I do not know. At fifteen she was an actress, determined to do her best, and ambitious of success. She strenuously taxed muscle and brain at all times in her calling. She worked in a man's sustained way, ignoring all demands for special development, and essaying first to dis-establish, and then to bridle, the catamenia. At twenty she was eminent. The excitement and effort of acting periodically produced the same result with her that a recitation did under similar conditions with Miss A——. If she had been a physiologist, she would have known how this course of action would end. As she was an actress, and not a physiologist, she persisted in the slow suicide of frequent hemorrhages, and encouraged them by her method of professional education, and later by her method of practising her profession. She tried to ward off disease, and repair the loss of force, by consulting various doctors, taking drugs, and resorting to all sorts of expedients ; but the hemorrhages continued, and were repeated at irregular and abnormally frequent intervals. A careful local examination disclosed no local disturbance. There was neither ulceration, hypertrophy, or congestion of the os or cervix uteri; no displacement of any moment, or ovarian tenderness. In spite of all her difficulties, however, she worked on courageously and steadily in a man's way and with a woman's will. After a long and discouraging experience of doctors, work, and weaknesses, when rather over thirty years old, she came to Boston to consult the writer, who learned at that time the details just recited. She was then pale and weak. A murmur in the veins, which a French savant, by way of dedication to the Devil, christened *bruit de diable*, a baptismal name that science has retained, was audible over her jugulars, and a similar murmur over her heart. Palpitation and labored respiration accompanied and impeded effort. She complained most of her head, which felt " queer," would not go to sleep as formerly, and often gave her turns, in which there was a mingling of dizziness, semi-consciousness, and fear. Her education and work, or rather method of work, had wrought out for her anemia and epileptiform attacks. She got two or three physiological lectures, was ordered to take iron, and other nourishing food, allow time for sleep, and, above all, to arrange her professional work in harmony with the rythmical or periodical action of woman's constitution. She made the effort to do this, and, in six months, reported herself in better health — though far from well — than she had been for six years before.

This case scarcely requires analysis in order to see how it bears on the question of a girl's education and woman's work. A gifted and healthy girl, obliged to get her education and earn her bread at the same time, labored upon the two tasks zealously, perhaps over-much, and did this at the epoch when the female organization is busy with the development of its reproductive apparatus. Nor is this all. She labored continuously, yielding nothing to Nature's periodical demand for force. She worked her engine up to highest pressure, just as much at flood-tide as at other times. Naturally there was not nervous power enough developed in the uterine and assaciated ganglia to restrain the laboring orifices of the circulation, to close the gates; and the flood of blood gushed through. With the frequent repetition of the flooding, came inevitably the evils she suffered from, — Nature's penalties. She now reports herself better; but whether convalescence will continue will depend upon her method of work for the future.

Let us take the next illustration from a walk in life different from either of the foregoing. Miss C——was a bookkeeper in a mercantile house. The length of time she remained in the employ of the house, and its character, are a sufficient guaranty that she did her work well. Like the other clerks, she was at her post, *standing*, during business hours, from Monday morning till Saturday night. The female pelvis being wider than that of the male, the weight of the body, in the upright posture, tends to press the upper extremities of the thighs out laterally in females more than in males. Hence the former can stand less long with comfort than the latter. Miss C——, however, believed in doing her

work in a man's way, infected by the not uncommon notion that womanliness means manli-
ness. Moreover, she would not, or could not,
make any more allowance for the periodicity
of her organization than for the shape of her
skeleton. When about twenty years of age,
perhaps a year or so older, she applied to me
for advice in consequence of neuralgia, back-
ache, menorrhagia, leucorrhœa, and general
debility. She was anemic, and looked pale,
care-worn, and anxious. There was no evidence of any local organic affection of the
pelvic organs. " Get a woman's periodical
remission from labor, if intermission is impossible, and do your work in a woman's way,
not copying a man's fashion, and you will
need very little apothecary's stuff," was the
advice she received. " I *must* go on as I am
doing," was her answer. She tried iron, sitz-
baths, and the like : of course they were of no
avail. Latterly I have lost sight of her, and,
from her appearance at her last visit to me,
presume she has gone to a world where back-
ache and male and female skeletons are unknown.

Illustrations of this sort might be multiplied; but these three are sufficient to show how an abnormal method of study and work may and does open the flood-gates of the system, and, by letting blood out, lets all sorts of evil in. Let us now look at another phase; for menorrhagia and its consequences are not the only punishments that girls receive for being educated and worked just like boys. Nature's methods of punishing men and women are as numerous as their organs and functions, and her penalties as infinite in number and gradation as her blessings.

Amenorrhœa is perhaps more common than menorrhagia. It often happens, however, during the first critical epoch, which is isochronal with the technical educational period of a girl, that after a few occasions of catamenial hemorrhage, moderate perhaps but still hemorrhage, which are not heeded, the conservative force of Nature steps in, and saves the blood by arresting the function. In such instances, amenorrhœa is a result of menorrhagia. In this way, and in others that we

need not stop to inquire into, the regimen of
our schools, colleges, and social life, that requires girls to walk, work, stand, study, recite,
and dance at all times as boys can and should,
may shut the uterine portals of the blood up,
and keep poison in, as well as open them, and
let life out. Which of these two evils is
worse in itself, and which leaves the largest
legacy of ills behind, it is difficult to say.
Let us examine some illustrations of this sort
of arrest.

Miss D—— entered Vassar College at the
age of fourteen. Up to that age, she had
been a healthy girl, judged by the standard
of American girls. Her parents were appar-
ently strong enough to yield her a fair dower
of force. The catamenial function first
showed signs of activity in her Sophomore
Year, when she was fifteen years old. Its
appearance at this age * is confirmatory evi-

* It appears, from the researches of Mr. Whitehead on
this point, that an examination of four thousand cases gave
fifteen years six and three-quarter months as the average
age in England for the appearance of the catamenia.—
WHITEHEAD, *on Abortion, &c.*

dence of the normal state of her health at that period of her college career. Its commencement was normal, without pain or excess. She performed all her college duties regularly and steadily. She studied, recited, stood at the blackboard, walked, and went through her gymnastic exercises, from the beginning to the end of the term, just as boys do. Her account of her regimen there was so nearly that of a boy's regimen, that it would puzzle a physiologist to determine, from the account alone, whether the subject of it was male or female. She was an average scholar, who maintained a fair position in her class, not one of the anxious sort, that are ambitious of leading all the rest. Her first warning was fainting away, while exercising in the gymnasium, at a time when she should have been comparatively quiet, both mentally and physically. This warning was repeated several times, under the same circumstances. Finally she was compelled to renounce gymnastic exercises altogether. In her Junior Year. the organism's periodical function began to be performed with pain, moderate at first, but more and more severe with each returning month. When between seventeen and eighteen years old, dysmenorrhœa was established as the order of that function. Coincident with the appearance of pain, there was a diminution of excretion; and, as the former increased, the latter became more marked. In other respects she was well; and, in all respects, she appeared to be well to her companions and to the faculty of the college. She graduated before nineteen, with fair honors and a poor physique. The year succeeding her graduation was one of steadily-advancing invalidism. She was tortured for two or three days out of every month; and, for two or three days after each season of torture, was weak and miserable, so that about one sixth or fifth of her time was consumed in this way. The excretion from the blood, which had been gradually lessening, after a time substantially stopped, though a periodical effort to keep it up was made. She now suffered

6

from what is called amenorrhœa. At the same time she became pale, hysterical, nervous in the ordinary sense, and almost constantly complained of headache. Physicians were applied to for aid: drugs were administered; travelling, with consequent change of air and scene, was undertaken; and all with little apparent avail. After this experience, she was brought to Boston for advice, when the writer first saw her, and learned all these details. She presented no evidence of local uterine congestion, inflammation, ulceration, or displacement. The evidence was altogether in favor of an arrest of the development of the reproductive apparatus, at a stage when the development was nearly complete. Confirmatory proof of such an arrest was found in examining her breast, where the milliner had supplied the organs Nature should have grown. It is unnecessary for our present purpose to detail what treatment was advised. It is sufficient to say, that she probably never will become physically what she would have been had her education being physiologically guided.

This case needs very little comment : its teachings are obvious. Miss D—— went to college in good physical condition. During the four years of her college life, her parents and the college faculty required her to get what is popularly called an education. Nature required her, during the same period, to build and put in working-order a large and complicated reproductive mechanism, a matter that is popularly ignored, — shoved out of sight like a disgrace. She naturally obeyed the requirements of the faculty, which she could see, rather than the requirements of the mechanism within her, that she could not see. Subjected to the college regimen, she worked four years in getting a liberal education. Her way of work was sustained and continuous, and out of harmony with the rhythmical periodicity of the female organization. The stream of vital and constructive force evolved within her was turned steadily to the brain, and away from the ovaries and their accessories. The result of this sort of education was, that these last-mentioned organs,

deprived of sufficient opportunity and nutriment, first began to perform their functions
with pain, a warning of error that was un-
heeded; then, to cease to grow ; * next, to set
up once a month a grumbling torture that
made life miserable ; and, lastly, the brain
and the whole nervous system, disturbed, in
obedience to the law, that, if one member
suffers, all the members suffer, became neuralgic and hysterical. And so Miss D——
spent the few years next succeeding her
graduation in conflict with dysmenorrhœa,
headache, neuralgia, and hysteria. Her
parents marvelled at her ill-heath; and she

---

* The arrest of development of the uterus, in connection
with amenorrhœa, is sometimes very marked. In the New-
York Medical Journal for June, 1873, three such cases are
recorded, that came under the eye of those excellent observers, Dr. E. R. Peaslee and Dr. T. G. Thomas. In one
of these cases, the uterine cavity measured one and a half
inches; in another, one and seven-eighths inches; and, in a
third, one and a quarter inches. Recollecting that the normal
measurement is from two and a half to three inches, it appears that the arrest of development in these cases occurred
when the uterus was half or less than half grown. Liberal
education should avoid such errors.

furnished another text for the often-repeated sermon on the delicacy of American girls.

It may not be unprofitable to give the history of one more case of this sort. Miss E—— had an hereditary right to a good brain and to the best cultivation of it. Her father was one of our ripest and broadest American scholars, and her mother one of our most accomplished American women. They both enjoyed excellent health. Their daughter had a literary training, — an intellectual, moral, and æsthetic half of education, such as their supervision would be likely to give, and one that few young men of her age receive. Her health did not seem to suffer at first. She studied, recited, walked, worked, stood, and the like, in the steady and sustained way that is normal to the male organization. She *seemed* to evolve force enough to acquire a number of languages, to become familiar with the natural sciences, to take hold of philosophy and mathematics, and to keep in good physical case while doing all this. At the age of

twenty-one she might have been presented
to the public, on Commencement Day, by the
president of Vassar College or of Antioch
College or of Michigan University, as the
wished-for result of American liberal female
culture. Just at this time, however, the
catamenial function began to show signs of
failure of power. No severe or even moderate illness overtook her. She was subjected
to no unusual strain. She was only following the regimen of continued and sustained
work, regardless of Nature's periodical demands for a portion of her time and force,
when, without any apparent cause, the failure of power was manifested by moderate
dysmenorrhœa and diminished excretion.
Soon after this the function ceased altogether; and up to this present writing, a period
of six or eight years, it has shown no more
signs of activity than an amputated arm.
In the course of a year or so after the cessa-
tion of the function, her head began to
trouble her. First there was headache, then
a frequent congested condition, which she

described as a " rush of blood " to her head ; and, by and by, vagaries and forebodings and despondent feelings began to crop out. Coincident with this mental state, her skin became rough and coarse, and an inveterate acne covered her face. She retained her appetite, ability to exercise and sleep. A careful local examination of the pelvic organs, by an expert, disclosed no lesion or displacement there, no ovaritis or other inflammation. Appropriate treatment faithfully persevered in was unsuccessful in recovering the lost function. I was finally obliged to consign her to an asylum.

The arrest of development of the reproductive system is most obvious to the superficial observer in that part of it which the milliner is called upon to cover up with pads, and which was alluded to in the case of Miss D——. This, however, is too important a matter to be dismissed with a bare allusion. A recent writer has pointed out the fact and its significance with great clearness. "There is another marked charge," says Dr. Nathan Allen, "going on in the female organization at the present day, which is very significant of something wrong. In the normal state, Nature has made ample provision in the structure of the female for nursing her offspring. In order to furnish this nourishment, pure in quality and abundant in quantity, she must possess a good development of the sanguine and lymphatic temperament, together with vigorous and healthy digestive organs. Formerly such an organization was very generally possessed by American women, and they found but little difficulty in nursing their infants. It was only occasionally, in case of some defect in the organization, or where sickness of some kind had overtaken the mother, that it became necessary to resort to the wet-nurse or to feeding by hand. And the English, the Scotch, the German, the Canadian French, and the Irish women now living in this country, generally nurse their children: the exceptions are rare. But how is it with our American women who become mothers? To those who have never considered this subject, and even to medical men who have never carefully looked into it, the facts, when correctly and fully presented, will be surprising. It has been supposed by some that all, or nearly all, our American women could nurse their offspring just as well as not; that the disposition only was wanting, and that they did not care about having the trouble or confinement necessarily attending it. But this is a great mistake. This very indifference or aversion shows something wrong in the organization as well as in the disposition : if the physical system were all right, the mind and natural instincts would generally be right also. While there may be here and there cases of this kind, such an indisposition is not always found. It is a fact, that large numbers of our women are anxious to nurse their offspring, and make the attempt : they persevere for a while, — perhaps for weeks or months, — and then fail. . . . There is still another class that cannot nurse at all, *having neither the organs nor nourishment* requisite even to make a beginning. . . . Why should there be such a difference between the women of our times and their mothers or grand-mothers? Why should there be such a dif-ference between our American women and those of foreign origin residing in the same locality, and surrounded by the same exter-nal influences? The explanation is simple: they have not the right kind of organization; there is a want of proper development of the lymphatic and sanguine temperaments, — a marked deficiency in the organs of nutrition and secretion. You cannot draw water without good, flowing springs. *The brain and nervous system have, for a long time, made relatively too large a demand upon* the organs of digestion and assimilation, while the exer-cise and *development of certain other tissues in the body have been sadly neglected.* . . . In consequence of the great neglect of physical exercise, and the *continuous application to study*, together with various other influences, large numbers of our American women have

altogether an undue predominance of the
nervous temperament. If only here and
there an individual were found with such an
organization, not much harm comparatively
would result; but, when a majority or nearly
all have it, the evil becomes one of no small
magnitude." *   And the evil, it should be
added, is not simply the inability to nurse; for,
if one member suffers, all the members suffer.
A woman, whether married or unmarried,
whether called to the offices of maternity or
relieved from them, who has been defrauded
by her education or otherwise of such an
essential part of her development, is not so
much of a woman, intellectually and morally
as well as physically, in consequence of this
defect.   Her nervous system and brain, her
instincts and character, are on a lower plane,
and incapable of their harmonious and best
development, if she is possessed, on reaching adult age, of only a portion of a breast
and an ovary, or none at all.

* Physical Degeneracy. By Nathan Allen, M.D., Journal
of Psychological Medicine.   October, 1870.

When arrested development of the reproductive system is nearly or quite complete, it produces a change in the character, and a loss of power, which it is easy to recognize, but difficult to describe. As this change is an occasional attendant or result of amenorrhœa, when the latter, brought about at an early age, is part of an early arrest, it should not be passed by without an allusion. In these cases, which are not of frequent occurrence at present, but which may be evolved by our methods of education more numerously in the future, the system tolerates the absence of the catamenia, and the consequent non-elimination of impurities from the blood. Acute or chronic disease, the ordinary result of this condition, is not set up, but, instead, there is a change in the character and development of the brain and nervous system. There are in individuals of this class less adipose and more muscular tissue than is commonly seen, a coarser skin, and, generally, a tougher and more angular make-up. There is a corresponding change in the intellectual and psychical condition, — a dropping out of maternal instincts, and an appearance of Amazonian coarseness and force. Such persons are analogous to the sexless class of termites. Naturalists tell us that these insects are divided into males and females, and a third class called workers and soldiers, who have no reproductive apparatus, and who, in their structure and instincts, are unlike the fertile individuals.

A closer analogy than this, however, exists between these human individuals and the eunuchs of Oriental civilization. Except the secretary of the treasury, in the cabinet of Candace, queen of Ethiopia, who was baptized by Philip and Narses, Justinian's general, none of that class have made any impression on the world's life, that history has recorded. It may be reasonably doubted if arrested development of the female reproductive system, producing a class of agenes,* not epicenes, will yield a

---

* According to the biblical account, woman was formed by subtracting a rib from man. If, in the evolution of the future, a third division of the human race is to be formed by subtracting sex from woman, — a retrograde development, —

better result of intellectual and moral power in the nineteenth century, than the analogous class of Orientals exhibited. Clinical illustrations of this type of arrested growth might be given, but my pen refuses the ungracious task.

Another result of the present methods of educating girls, and one different from any of the preceding, remains to be noticed. Schools and colleges, as we have seen, require girls to work their brains with full force and sustained power, at the time when their organization periodically requires a portion of their force for the performance of a periodical function, and a portion of their power for the building up of a peculiar, complicated, and important mechanism, — the engine within an engine. They are required to do two

---

I venture to propose the term agene (*a* without, *γενος* sex) as an appropriate designation for the new development. Count Gasparin prophesies it thus : " Quelque chose de monstreux, cet être répugnant, qui déjà parait à notre horizon," a free translation of Virgil's earlier description : —

"Monstrum horrendum, informe, ingens, cui lumen ademtum."
3*d*, 658 *line.*

things equally well at the same time. They are urged to meditate a lesson and drive a machine simultaneously, and to do them both with all their force. Their organizations are expected to make good sound brains and nerves by working over the humanities, the sciences, and the arts, and, at the same time, to make good sound reproductive apparatuses, not only without any especial attention to the latter, but while all available force is withdrawn from the latter and sent to the former. It is not materialism to say, that, as the brain is, so will thought be. Without discussing the French physiologist's dictum, that the brain secretes thought as the liver does bile, we may be sure, that without brain there will be no thought. The quality of the latter depends on the quality of the former. The metamorphoses of brain manifest, measure, limit, enrich, and color thought. Brain tissue, including both quantity and quality, correlates mental power. The brain is manufactured from the blood ; its quantity **and quality** are determined by the quantity

and quality of its blood supply. Blood is
made from food; but it may be lost by careless hemorrhage, or poisoned by deficient elimination. When frequently and largely lost
or poisoned, as I have too frequent occasion
to know it often is, it becomes impoverished,
— anemic. Then the brain suffers, and mental power is lost. The steps are few and
direct, from frequent loss of blood, impoverished blood, and abnormal brain and
nerve metamorphosis, to loss of mental force
and nerve disease. Ignorance or carelessness
leads to anemic blood, and that to an anemic
mind. As the blood, so the brain; as the
brain, so the mind.

The cases which have hitherto been presented illustrate some of the evils which the
reproductive system is apt to receive in consequence of obvious derangement of its
growth and functions. But it may, and often
does, happen that the catamenia are normally
performed, and that the reproductive system
is fairly made up during the educational
period. Then force is withdrawn from the

brain and nerves and ganglia. These are dwarfed or checked or arrested in their development. In the process of waste and repair, of destructive and constructive metamorphosis, by which brains as well as bones are built up and consolidated, education often leaves insufficient margin for growth Income derived from air, food, and sleep, which should largely, may only moderately exceed expenditure upon study and work, and so leave but little surplus for growth in any direction; or, what more commonly occurs, the income which the brain receives is all spent upon study, and little or none upon its development, while that which the nutritive and reproductive systems receive is retained by them, and devoted to their own growth. When the school makes the same steady demand for force from girls who are approaching puberty, ignoring Nature's periodical demands, that it does from boys, who are not called upon for an equal effort, there must be failure somewhere. Generally either the reproductive

7

system or the nervous system suffers. We
have looked at several instances of the former sort of failure ; let us now examine some
of the latter.

Miss F——— was about twenty years old
when she completed her technical education.
She inherited a nervous diathesis as well as a
large dower of intellectual and æsthetic
graces. She was a good student, and con-
scientiously devoted all her time, with the
exception of ordinary vacations, to the labor
of her education. She made herself mistress
of several languages, and accomplished in
many ways. The catamenial function appeared normally, and, with the exception of
occasional slight attacks of menorrhagia,
was normally performed during the whole
period of her education. She got on without
any sort of serious illness. There were few
belonging to my clientele who required less
professional advice for the same period than
she. With the ending of her school life,
when she should have been in good trim and
well equipped, physically as well as intel-

lectually, for life's work, there commenced, without obvious cause, a long period of invalidism. It would be tedious to the reader, and useless for our present purpose, to detail the history and describe the protean shapes of her sufferings. With the exception of small breasts, the reproductive system was well developed. Repeated and careful examinations failed to detect any derangement of the uterine mechanism. Her symptoms all pointed to the nervous system as the *fons et origo mali*. First general debility, that concealed but ubiquitous leader of innumerable armies of weakness and ill, laid siege to her, and captured her. Then came insomnia, that worried her nights for month after month, and made her beg for opium, alcohol, chloral, bromides, any thing that would bring sleep. Neuralgia in every conceivable form tormented her, most frequently in her back, but often, also, in her head, sometimes in her sciatic neives, sometimes setting up a tic douloureux, sometimes causing a fearful dysmenorrhœa and frequently making her head ache for days together. At other times hysteria got hold of her, and made her fancy herself the victim of strange diseases. Mental effort of the slightest character distressed her, and she could not bear physical exercise of any amount. This condition, or rather these varying conditions, continued for some years. She followed a careful and systematic regimen, and was rewarded by a slow and gradual return of health and strength, when a sudden accident killed her, and terminated her struggle with weakness and pain.

Words fail to convey the lesson of this case to others with any thing like the force that the observation of it conveyed its moral to those about Miss F——, and especially to the physician who watched her career through her educational life, and saw it lead to its logical conclusion of invalidism and thence towards recovery, till life ended. When she finished school, as the phrase goes, she was considered to be well. The principal of any seminary or head of any college, judging by her looks alone, would not have hesitated to call her rosy and strong. At that time the symptoms of failure which began to appear were called signs of previous overwork. This was true, but not so much in the sense of overwork as of erroneously-arranged work. While a student, she wrought continuously, — just as much during each catamenial week as at other times. As a consequence, in her metamorphosis of tissue, repair did little more than make up waste. There were constant demands of force for constant growth of the system generally, equally constant demands of force for the labor of education, and periodical demands of force for a periodical function. The regimen she followed did not permit all these demands to be satisfied, and the failure fell on the nervous system. She accomplished intellectually a good deal, but not more than she might have done, and retained her health, had the order of her education been a physiological one. It was not Latin, French, German, mathematics, or

philosophy that undermined her nerves; nor
was it because of any natural inferiority to
boys that she failed; nor because she undertook to master what women have no right to
learn : she lost her health simply because
she undertook to do her work in a boy's way
and not in a girl's way.

Let us learn the lesson of one more case.
These details may be tedious; but the justi-
fication of their presence here are the importance of the subject they illustrate and
elucidate, and the necessity of acquiring a
belief of the truth of the facts of female
education.

Miss G—— worked her way through New-
England primary, grammar, and high schools
to a Western college, which she entered with
credit to herself, and from which she graduated, confessedly its first scholar, leading the
male and female youth alike. All that need
be told of her career is that she worked as
a student, continuously and perseveringly,
through the years of her first critical epoch,
and for a few years after it, without any

sort of regard to the periodical type of her
organization. It never appeared that she
studied excessively in other respects, or that
her system was weakened while in college
by fevers or other sickness. Not a great
while after graduation, she began to show
signs of failure, and some years later died
under the writer's care. A post-mortem ex
amination was made, which disclosed no dis
ease in any part of the body, except in the
brain, where the microscope revealed com-
mencing degeneration.

This was called an instance of death from
over-work. Like the preceding case, it was
not so much the result of over-work as of
un-physiological work. She was unable to
make a good brain, that could stand the
wear and tear of life, and a good reproductive system that should serve the race,
at the same time that she was continuously
spending her force in intellectual labor.
Nature asked for a periodical remission,
and did not get it. And so Miss G——
died, not because she had mastered the

wasps of Aristophanes and the Mécanique Céleste, not because she had made the acquaintance of Kant and Kölliker, and ventured to explore the anatomy of flowers and the secrets of chemistry, but because, while pursuing these studies, while doing all this work, she steadily ignored her woman's make. Believing that woman can do what man can, for she held that faith, she strove with noble but ignorant bravery to compass man's intellectual attainment in a man's way, and died in the effort. If she had aimed at the same goal, disregarding masculine and following feminine methods, she would be alive now, a grand example of female culture, attainment, and power.

These seven clinical observations are sufficient to illustrate the fact that our modern methods of education do not give the female organization a fair chance, but that they check development, and invite weakness. It would be easy to multiply such observations, from the writer's own notes alone, and, by doing so, to swell this essay into a portly volume; but the reader is spared the needless infliction. Other observers have noticed similar facts, and have urgently called attention to them.

Dr. Fisher, in a recent excellent monograph on insanity, says, " A few examples of injury from *continued* study will show how mental strain affects the health of young girls particularly. Every physician could, no doubt, furnish many similar ones."

" Miss A—— graduated with honor at the normal school after several years of close study, much of the time out of school; never attended balls or parties; sank into a low state of health at once with depression. Was very absurdly allowed to marry while in this state, and soon after became violently insane, and is likely to remain so."

" Miss A—— graduated at the grammar school, not only first, but *perfect*, and at once entered the normal school; was very ambitious to sustain her reputation, and studied hard out of school; was slow to learn, but had a retentive memory; could seldom be induced to go to parties, and, when she did go, studied while dressing, and on the way; was assigned extra tasks at school, because she performed them so well; was a *fine healthy girl in appearance*, but broke down permanently at end of second year, and is now a victim of hysteria and depression."

" Miss C——, of a nervous organization, and quick to learn; her health suffered in normal school, so that her physician predicted insanity if her studies were not discontinued. She persevered, however, and is now an inmate of a hospital, with hysteria and depression."

" A certain proportion of girls are predisposed to mental or nervous derangement. The same girls are apt to be quick, brilliant, ambitious, and persistent at study, and need not stimulation, but repression. For the sake of a temporary reputation for scholarship, they risk their health at the *most susceptible period* of their lives, and break down *after the excitement of school-life has passed away.* For *sexual reasons* they cannot compete with boys, whose out-door habits still further increase the difference in their favor. If it was a question of school-teachers instead of school-girls, the list would be long of young women whose health of mind has become bankrupt by a *continuation* of the mental strain commenced at school. Any method of relief in our school-system to these over-susceptible minds should be welcomed, even at the cost of the intellectual supremacy of woman in the next generation." *

The fact which Dr. Fisher alludes to, that many girls break down not during but *after* the excitement of school or college life, is an important one, and is apt to be overlooked. The process by which the development of the reproductive system is arrested, or degeneration of brain and nerve-tissue set a going, is an insidious one. At its beginning, and for a long time after it is well on in its progress, it would not be recognized by the superficial observer. A class of girls might, and often

---

* Plain Talk about Insanity. By T. W. Fisher, M.D. Boston. Pp. 23, 24.

do, graduate from our schools, higher seminaries, and colleges, that appear to be well and
strong at the time of their graduation, but
whose development has already been checked,
and whose health is on the verge of giving
way.   Their teachers have known nothing
of the amenorrhœa, menorrhagia, dysmenorrhœa, or leucorrhœa which the pupils have
sedulously concealed and disregarded; and the
cunning devices of dress have covered up all
external evidences of defect; and so, on
graduation day, they are pointed out by their
instructors to admiring committees as rosy
specimens of both physical and intellectual
education.   A closer inspection by competent
experts would reveal the secret weakness
which the labor of life that they are about
to enter upon too late discloses.

The testimony of Dr. Anstie of London, as
to the gravity of the evils incurred by the
sort of erroneous education we are considering, is decided and valuable.   He says, " For,
be it remembered, the epoch of sexual development is one in which an enormous addition

is being made to the expenditure of vital energy; besides the continuous processes of
growth of the tissues and organs generally,
the sexual apparatus, with its nervous supply,
is making *by its development heavy demands*
upon the nutritive powers of the organism;
and it is scarcely possible but that portions of
the nervous centres, not directly connected
with it, should proportionally suffer in their
nutrition, probably through defective blood
supply. When we add to this the abnormal
strain that is being put on the brain, in many
cases, by a forcing plan of mental education, we
shall perceive a source not merely of exhaust-
ive expenditure of nervous power, but of sec-
ondary irritation of centres like the medulla
oblongata that are probably already somewhat
lowered in power of vital resistance, and pro-
portionably *irritable*." *   A little farther on,
Dr. Anstie adds, " But I confess, that, with
me, the result of close attention given to the
pathology of neuralgia has been the ever-

* Neuralgia, and the Diseases that resemble it. By Fran-
cis E. Anstie, M.D.   Pp. 122.   English ed.

growing conviction, that, next to the influence of neurotic inheritance, there is no such frequently powerful factor in the construction of the neuralgic habit as mental warp of a certain kind, the product of an unwise education." In another place, speaking of the liability of the brain to suffer from an unwise education, and referring to the sexual development that we are discussing in these pages, he makes the following statement, which no intelligent physician will deny, and which it would be well for all teachers who care for the best education of the girls intrusted to their charge to ponder seriously. " I would also go farther, and express the opinion, that peripheral influences of an extremely powerful and *continuous* kind, where they concur with one of those critical periods of life at which the central nervous system is relatively weak and unstable, can occasionally set going a non-inflammatory centric atrophy, which may localize itself in those nerves upon whose centres the morbific peripheral influence is perpetually pouring in. Even such influences as the psy-

chical and emotional, be it remembered, must
be considered peripheral." * The brain of
Miss G——, whose case was related a few
pages back, is a clinical illustration of the
accuracy of this opinion.

Dr. Weir Mitchell, one of our most eminent
American physiologists, has recently borne
most emphatic testimony to the evils we have
pointed out : " Worst of all," he says, " to my
mind, most destructive in every way, is the
American view of female education. The
time taken for the more serious instruction of
girls extends to the age of eighteen, and
rarely over this. During these years, they
are undergoing such organic development as
renders them remarkably sensitive." . . . " To
show more precisely how the growing girl is
injured by the causes just mentioned " (forced
and continued study at the sexual epoch)
" would carry me upon subjects unfit for full
discussion in these pages ; but no thoughtful
reader can be much at a loss as to my mean-
ing." . . . " To-day the American woman is,

---

* Op. cit., p. 160.

to speak plainly, physically unfit for her duties as woman, and is, perhaps, of all civilized females, the least qualified to undertake those weightier tasks which tax so heavily the nervous system of man. She is not fairly up to what Nature asks from her as wife and mother. How will she sustain herself under the pressure of those yet more exacting duties which now-a-days she is eager to share with the man ? " *

In our schools it is the ambitious and conscientious girls, those who have in them the stuff of which the noblest women are made, that suffer, not the romping or lazy sort ; and thus our modern ways of education provide for the " non-survival of the fittest." A speaker told an audience of women at Wesleyan Hall not long ago, that he once attended the examination of a Western college, where a girl beat the boys in unravelling the intracacies of Juvenal. He did not report the consumption of blood and wear of brain tissue that in her college way of study correlated

---

* Wear and Tear. By S. Weir Mitchell, M.D.

her Latin, or hint at the possibility of arrested development. Girls of bloodless skins and intellectual faces may be seen any day, by those who desire the spectacle, among the scholars of our high and normal schools, — faces that crown, and skins that cover, curving spines, which should be straight, and neuralgic nerves that should know no pain. Later on, when marriage and maternity overtake these girls, and they "live laborious days" in a sense not intended by Milton's line, they bend and break beneath the labor, like loaded grain before a storm, and bear little fruit again. A training that yields this result is neither fair to the girls nor to the race.

Let us quote the authority of such an acute and sagacious observer as Dr. Maudsley, in support of the physiological and pathological views that have been here presented. Referring to the physiological condition and phenomena of the first critical epoch, he says, "In the great mental revolution caused by the development of the sexual system at puberty, we have the most striking example of the

8

intimate and essential sympathy between the brain, as a mental organ, and other organs of the body. The change of character at this period is not by any means *limited to the appearance of the sexual feelings,* and their sympathetic ideas, but, when traced to its ultimate reach, will be found to extend to the highest feelings of mankind, social, moral, and even religious." *   He points out the fact that it is very easy by improper training and forced work, during this susceptible period, to turn a physiological into a pathological state.   " The great mental revolution which occurs at puberty may go beyond its physiological limits in some instances, and become pathological."   " The time of this mental revolution is at best a trying period for youth." " The monthly activity of the ovaries, which marks the advent of puberty in women, has a notable effect upon the mind and body ; wherefore it may become an important cause of mental and physical derangement." †

* Body and Mind.   By Henry Maudsley, M.D.   Lond. p. 31.
† Op. cit., p. 87.

With regard to the physiological effects of arrested development of the reproductive apparatus in women, Dr. Maudsley uses the following plain and emphatic language : " The forms and habits of mutilated men approach those of women ; and women, whose ovaries and uterus remain for some cause in a state of complete inaction, approach the forms and habits of men. It is said, too, that, in hermaphrodites, the mental character, like the physical, participates equally in that of both sexes. While woman preserves her sex, she will necessarily be feebler than man, and, having her special bodily and mental characters, will have, to a certain extent, her own sphere of activity ; where she has become thoroughly masculine in nature, or hermaphrodite in mind, — when, in fact, she has pretty well divested herself of her sex, — then she may take his ground, and do his work ; but she will have lost her feminine attractions, and probably also her chief feminine functions." *

---

* Op. cit., p. 32.

It has been reserved for our age and country, by its methods of female education, to demonstrate that it is possible in some cases to divest a woman of her chief feminine functions ; in others, to produce grave and even fatal disease of the brain and nervous system ; in others, to engender torturing derangements and imperfections of the reproductive apparatus that imbitter a lifetime. Such, we know, is not the object of a liberal female education. Such is not the consummation which the progress of the age demands. Fortunately, it is only necessary to point out and prove the existence of such erroneous methods and evil results to have them avoided. That they can be avoided, and that woman can have a liberal education that shall develop all her powers, without mutilation or disease, up to the loftiest ideal of womanhood, is alike the teaching of physiology and the hope of the race.

In concluding this part of our subject, it is well to remember the statement made at the beginning of our discussion, to the fol-

lowing effect, viz., that it is not asserted
here, that improper methods of study and a
disregard of the reproductive apparatus and
its functions, during the educational life of
girls, are the *sole* causes of female diseases;
neither is it asserted that *all* the female graduates of our schools and colleges are pathological specimens. But it is asserted that the
number of these graduates who have been
permantly disabled to a greater or less degree,
or fatally injured, by these causes, is such as to
excite the *gravest alarm*, and to demand the
serious attention of the community.

The preceding physiological and pathological data naturally open the way to a consideration of the co-education of the sexes.

PART IV.

CO-EDUCATION.

" Pistoc. Where, then, should I take my place?

1*st Bacch.* Near myself, that, with a she wit, a he wit may
be reclining at our repast." — BACCHIDES OF PLAUTUS.

" The woman's-rights movement, with its conventions, its
speech-makings, its crudities, and eccentricities, is neverthe-
less a part of a healthful and necessary movement of the human race towards progress." — HARRIET BEECHER STOWE.

GUIDED by the laws of development which
we have found physiology to teach, and
warned by the punishments, in the shape of
weakness and disease, which we have shown
their infringement to bring about, and of
which our present methods of female education furnish innumerable examples, it is not
difficult to discern certain physiological principles that limit and control the education,
and, consequently, the co-education of our

youth. These principles we have learned to be, three for the two sexes in common, and one for the peculiarities of the female sex. The three common to both, the three to which both are subjected, and for which wise methods of education will provide in the case of both, are, 1st, a sufficient supply of appropriate nutriment. This of course includes good air and good water and sufficient warmth, as much as bread and butter ; oxygen and sunlight, as much as meat. 2d, Mental and physical work and regimen so apportioned, that repair shall exceed waste, and a margin be left for development. This includes out-of-door exercise and appropriate ways of dressing, as much as the hours of study, and the number and sort of studies. 3d, Sufficient sleep. This includes the best time for sleeping, as well as the proper number of hours for sleep. It excludes the " murdering of sleep," by late hours of study and the crowding of studies, as much as by wine or tea or dissipation. All these guide and limit the education of the two sexes very much alike. The principle or condition peculiar to the female sex is the management of the catamenial function, which, from the age of fourteen to nineteen, includes the building of the reproductive apparatus. This imposes upon women, and especially upon the young woman, a great care, a corresponding duty, and compensating privileges. There is only a feeble counterpart to it in the male organization ; and, in his moral constitution, there cannot be found the fine instincts and quick perceptions that have their root in this mechanism, and correlate its functions. This lends to her development and to all her work a rythmical or periodical order, which must be recognized and obeyed.   " In this recognition of the chronometry of organic process, there is unquestionably great promise for the future ; for it is plain that the observance of time in the motions of organic molecules is as certain and universal, if not as exact, as that of the heavenly bodies." *   Periodicity characterizes the female organization,

---

* Body and Mind.   Op. cit., p. 178.

and developes feminine force. Persistence characterizes the male organization, and develops masculine force. Education will draw the best out of each by adjusting its methods to the periodicity of one and the persistence of the other.

Before going farther, it is essential to acquire a definite notion of what is meant, or, at least, of what we mean in this discussion, by the term co-education. Following its etymology, *con-educare*, it signifies to draw out together, or to unite in education ; and this union refers to the time and place, rather than to the methods and kinds of education. In this sense any school or college may utilize its buildings, apparatus, and instructors to give appropriate education to the two sexes as well as to different ages of the same sex. This is juxtaposition in education. When the Massachusetts Institute of Technology teaches one class of young men chemistry, and another class engineering, in the same building and at the same time, it co-educates those two classes. In this sense it is possible that many advantages might be obtained from the co-education of the sexes, that would more than counterbalance the evils of crowding large numbers of them together. This sort of co-education does not exclude appropriate classification, nor compel the two sexes to follow the same methods or the same regimen.

Another signification of co-education, and, as we apprehend, the one in which it is commonly used, includes time, place, government, methods, studies, and regimen. This is identical co-education. This means, that boys and girls shall be taught the same things, at the same time, in the same place, by the same faculty, with the same methods, and under the same regimen. This admits age and proficiency, but not sex, as a factor in classification. It is against the co-education of the sexes, in this sense of identical co-education, that physiology protests; and it is this identity of education, the prominent characteristic of our American school-system, that has produced the evils described in the clinical part of this essay, and that threatens to push the degeneration of the female sex still farther on. In these pages, co-education of the sexes is used in its common acceptation of identical co-education.

Let us look for a moment at what identical co-education is. The law has, or had, a maxim, that a man and his wife are one, and that the one is the man. Modern American education has a maxim, that boys' schools and girls' schools are one, and that the one is the boys' school. Schools have been arranged, accordingly, to meet the requirements of the masculine organization. Studies have been selected that experience has proved to be appropriate to a boy's intellectual development, and a regimen adopted, while pursuing them, appropriate to his physical development. His school and college life, his methods of study, recitations, exercises, and recreations, are ordered upon the supposition, that, barring disease or infirmity, punctual attendance upon the hours of recitation, and upon all other duties in their season and order, may be required of him continuously, in

spite of ennui, inclement weather, or fatigue ; that there is no week in the month,
or day in the week, or hour in the day,
when it is a physical necessity to relieve
him from standing or from studying, — from
physical effort or mental labor ; that the
chapel-bell may safely call him to morning
prayer from New Year to Christmas, with the
assurance, that, if the going does not add to
his stock of piety, it will not diminish his
stock of health ; that he may be sent to the
gymnasium and the examination-hall, to the
theatres of physical and intellectual display at
any time, — in short, that he develops health
and strength, blood and nerve, intellect and
life, by a regular, uninterrupted, and sustained
course of work.   And all this is justified both
by experience and physiology.

Obedient to the American educational
maxim, that boys' schools and girls' schools
are one, and that the one is the boys' school,
the female schools have copied the methods
which have grown out of the requirements of
the male organization.   Schools for girls have

been modelled after schools for boys. Were it not for differences of dress and figure, it would be impossible, even for an expert, after visiting a high school for boys and one for girls, to tell which was arranged for the male and which for the female organization. Our girls' schools, whether public or private, have imposed upon their pupils a boy's regimen ; and it is now proposed, in some quarters, to carry this principle still farther, by burdening girls, after they leave school, with a quadrennium of masculine college regimen. And so girls are to learn the alphabet in college, as they have learned it in the grammar-school, just as boys do. This is grounded upon the supposition that sustained regularity of action and attendance may be as safely required of a girl as of a boy ; that there is no physical necessity for periodically relieving her from walking, standing, reciting, or studying ; that the chapel-bell may call her, as well as him, to a daily morning walk, with a standing prayer at the end of it, regardless of the danger that such exercises, by deranging the tides of her organization, may add to her piety at the expense of her blood ; that she may work her brain over mathematics, botany, chemistry, German, and the like, with equal and sustained force on every day of the month, and so safely divert blood from the reproductive apparatus to the head ; in short, that she, like her brother, develops health and strength, blood and nerve, intellect and life, by a regular, uninterrupted, and sustained course of work.   All this is not justified, either by experience or physiology. The gardener may plant, if he choose, the lily and the rose, the oak and the vine, within the same enclosure ; let the same soil nourish them, the same air visit them, and the same sunshine warm and cheer them ; still, he trains each of them with a separate art, warding from each its peculiar dangers, developing within each its peculiar powers, and teaching each to put forth to the utmost its divine and peculiar gifts of strength and beauty. Girls lose health, strength, blood, and nerve, by a regimen that ignores the periodical tides and reproductive apparatus of their organization. The mothers and instructors, the homes and schools, of our country's daughters, would profit by occasionally reading the old Levitical law. The race has not yet quite outgrown the physiology of Moses.

Co-education, then, signifies in common acceptation identical co-education. This identity of training is what many at the present day seem to be praying for and working for. Appropriate education of the two sexes, carried as far as possible, is a consummation most devoutly to be desired; identical education of the two sexes is a crime before God and humanity, that physiology protests against, and that experience weeps over. Because the education of boys has met with tolerable success, hitherto, — but only tolerable it must be confessed, — in developing them into men, there are those who would make girls grow into women by the same process. Because a gardener has nursed an acorn till it grew into an oak, they would have him cradle a grape in the same soil and way, and make

it a vine.   Identical education, or identical
co-education, of the sexes defrauds one sex
or the other, or perhaps both.   It defies the
Roman maxim, which physiology has fully
justified, *mens sana in corpore sano.*   The
sustained regimen, regular recitation, erect
posture, daily walk, persistent exercise, and
unintermitted labor that toughens a boy, and
makes a man of him, can only be partially
applied to a girl.   The regimen of intermit-
tance, periodicity of exercise and rest, work
three-fourths of each month, and remission,
if not abstinence, the other fourth, physiological interchange of the erect and reclining
posture, care of the reproductive system that
is the cradle of the race, all this, that toughens a girl and makes a woman of her, will
emasculate a lad.   A combination of the two
methods of education, a compromise between
them, would probably yield an average result,
excluding the best of both.   It would give a
fair chance neither to a boy nor a girl.   Of all
compromises, such a physiological one is the
worst.   It cultivates mediocrity, and cheats

the future of its rightful legacy of lofty man
hood and womanhood. It emasculates boys,
stunts girls ; makes semi-eunuchs of one sex,
and agenes of the other.

The error which has led to the identical
education of the two sexes, and which proph-
ecies their identical co-education in colleges
and universities, is not confined to technical
education. It permeates society. It is
found in the home, the workshop, the
factory, and in all the ramifications of social
life. The identity of boys and girls, of men
and women, is practically asserted out of the
school as much as in it, and it is theoretically
proclaimed from the pulpit and the rostrum.
Woman seems to be looking up to man and
his development, as the goal and ideal of womanhood. The new gospel of female development glorifies what she possesses in common with him, and tramples under her feet,
as a source of weakness and badge of inferiority, the mechanism and functions peculiar
to herself. In consequence of this wide-
spread error, largely the result of physio-

logical ignorance, girls are almost universally trained in masculine methods of living and working as well as of studying. The notion is practically found everywhere, that boys and girls are one, and that the boys make the one. Girls, young ladies, to use the polite phrase, who are about leaving or have left school for society, dissipation, or self-culture, rarely permit any of Nature's periodical demands to interfere with their morning calls, or evening promenades, or midnight dancing, or sober study. Even the home draws the sacred mantle of modesty so closely over the reproductive function as not only to cover but to smother it. Sisters imitate brothers in persistent work at all times. Female clerks in stores strive to emulate the males by unremitting labor, seeking to develop feminine force by masculine methods. Female operatives of all sorts, in factories and elsewhere, labor in the same way; and, when the day is done, are as likely to dance half the night, regardless of any pressure upon them of a peculiar function, as their

fashionable sisters in the polite world. All
unite in pushing the hateful thing out of
sight and out of mind ; and all are punished
by similar weakness, degeneration, and
disease.

There are two reasons why female operatives of all sorts are likely to suffer less, and
actually do suffer less, from such persistent
work, than female students ; why Jane in
the factory can work more steadily with the
loom, than Jane in college with the dictionary ; why the girl who makes the bed can
safely work more steadily the whole year
through, than her little mistress of sixteen
who goes to school. The first reason is, that
the female operative, of whatever sort, has,
as a rule, passed through the first critical
epoch of woman's life : she has got fairly by
it. In her case, as a rule, unfortunately
there are too many exceptions to it, the catamenia have been established ; the function
is in good running order ; the reproductive apparatus — the engine within an engine — has been constructed, and she will

not be called upon to furnish force for building it again. The female student, on the
contrary, has got these tasks before her, and
must perform them while getting her education ; for the period of female sexual development coincides with the educational period.
The same five years of life must be given to
both tasks. After the function is normally
established, and the apparatus made, woman
can labor mentally or physically, or both,
with very much greater persistence and
intensity, than during the age of development. She still retains the type of periodicity ; and her best work, both as to quality
and amount, is accomplished when the order
of her labor partakes of the rhythmic order
of her constitution. Still the fact remains,
that she can do more than before ; her fibre
has acquired toughness ; the system is consolidated ; its fountains are less easily stirred.
It should be mentioned in this connection,
what has been previously adverted to, that
the toughness and power of after life are
largely in proportion to the normality of sex-

ual development. If there is error then, the organization never fully recovers. This is an additional motive for a strict physiological regimen during a girl's student life, and, just so far, an argument against the identical co-education of the sexes. The second reason why female operatives are less likely to suffer, and actually do suffer less, than school-girls, from persistent work straight through the year, is because the former work their brains less. To use the language of Herbert Spencer, " That antagonism between body and brain which we see in those, who, pushing brain-activity to an extreme, enfeeble their bodies," * does not often exist in female operatives, any more than in male. On the contrary, they belong to the class of those who, in the words of the same author, by " pushing bodily activity to an extreme, make their brains inert." * Hence they have stronger bodies, a reproductive apparatus more normally constructed, and a catamenial function less readily disturbed by effort, than

* The Study of Sociology, by Herbert Spencer, chap. 13.

their student sisters, who are not only younger than they, but are trained to push " brain-activity to an extreme." Give girls a fair chance for physical development at school, and they will be able in after life, with reasonable care of themselves, to answer the demands that may be made upon them.

The identical education of the sexes has borne the fruit which we have pointed out. Their identical co-education will intensify the evils of separate identical education; for it will introduce the element of emulation, and it will introduce this element in its strongest form. It is easy to frame a theoretical emulation, in which results only are compared and tested, that would be healthy and invigorating; but such theoretical competition of the sexes is not at all the sort of steady, untiring, day-after-day competition that identical co-education implies. It is one thing to put up a goal a long way off, — five or six months or three or four years distant, — and tell boys and girls, each in their own way, to strive for it, and quite a different thing to put up the same goal, at the same distance, and oblige each sex to run their race for it side by side on the same road, in daily competition with each other, and with equal expenditure of force at all times. Identical co-education is racing in the latter way. The inevitable results of it have been shown in some of the cases we have narrated. The trial of it on a larger scale would only yield a larger number of similar degenerations, weaknesses, and sacrifices of noble lives. Put a boy and girl together upon the same course of study, with the same lofty ideal before them, and hold up to their eyes the daily incitements of comparative progress, and there will be awakened within them a stimulus unknown before, and that separate study does not excite. The unconscious fires that have their seat deep down in the recesses of the sexual organization will flame up through every tissue, permeate every vessel, burn every nerve, flash from the eye, tingle in the brain, and work the whole machine at highest pressure. There need not be, and

generally will not be, any low or sensual
desire in all this elemental action. It is only
making youth work over the tasks of sober
study with the wasting force of intense pas-
sion. Of course such strenuous labor will
yield brilliant, though temporary, results.
The fire is kept alive by the waste of the
system, and soon burns up its source. The
first sex to suffer in this exhilarating and
costly competition must be, as experience
shows it is, the one that has the largest
amount of force in readiness for immediate
call ; and this is the female sex. At the age
of development, Nature mobilizes the forces
of a girl's organization for the purpose of
establishing a function that shall endure for
a generation, and for constructing an apparatus that shall cradle and nurse a race. These
mobilized forces, which, at the technical
educational period, the girl possesses and
controls largely in excess of the boy, under
the passionate stimulus of identical co-education, are turned from their divinely-appointed field of operations, to the region of

brain activity. The result is a most brilliant show of cerebral pyrotechnics, and degenerations that we have described.

That undue and disproportionate brain activity exerts a sterilizing influence upon both sexes is alike a doctrine of physiology, and an induction from experience. And both physiology and experience also teach that this influence is more potent upon the female than upon the male. The explanation of the latter fact — of the greater aptitude of the female organization to become thus modified by excessive brain activity — is probably to be found in the larger size, more complicated relations, and more important functions, of the female reproductive apparatus. This delicate and complex mechanism is liable to be aborted or deranged by the withdrawal of force that is needed for its construction and maintenance. It is, perhaps, idle to speculate upon the prospective evil that would accrue to the human race, should such an organic modification, introduced by abnormal education, be pushed to

its ultimate limit.   But inasmuch as the
subject is not only germain to our inquiry,
but has attracted the attention of a recent
writer, whose bold and philosophic specula-
tions, clothed in forcible language, have
startled the best thought of the age, it may
be well to quote him briefly on this point.
Referring to the fact, that, in our modern civilization, the cultivated classes have smaller
families than the uncultivated ones, he says,
" If the superior sections and specimens of
humanity are to lose, relatively, their procre-
ative power in virtue of, and in proportion to,
that superiority, how is culture or progress to
be propagated so as to benefit the species as
a whole, and how are those gradually
amended organizations from which we hope
so much to be secured ?   If, indeed, it were
ignorance, stupidity, and destitution, instead
of mental and moral development, that were
the *sterilizing* influences, then the improve-
ment of the race would go on swimmingly,
and in an ever-accelerating ratio.   But since
the conditions are exactly reversed, how

should not an exactly opposite direction be pursued ? How should the race *not* deteriorate, when those who morally and physically are fitted to perpetuate it are (relatively), by a law of physiology, those least likely to do so ? " * The answer to Mr. Greg's inquiry is obvious. If the culture of the race moves on into the future in the same rut and by the same methods that limit and direct it now ; if the education of the sexes remains identical, instead of being appropriate and special; and especially if the intense and passionate stimulus of the identical co-education of the sexes is added to their identical education,—then the sterilizing influence of such a training, acting with tenfold more force upon the female than upon the male, will go on, and the race will be propagated from its inferior classes.†

---

* Enigmas of Life. Op. cit., by **W. R.** Greg, p. 142.

† It is a fact not to be lost sight of, says **Dr. J. C. Toner** of Washington, that the proportion between the number of American children under fifteen years of age, and the number of American women between the child-bearing ages of fifteen and fifty, is declining steadily. In 1830, there were to every 1,000 marriageable women, 1,952 children under fifteen years

The stream of life that is to flow into the
future will be Celtic rather than American :
it will come from the collieries, and not from
the peerage. Fortunately, the reverse of this
picture is equally possible. The race holds
its destinies in its own hands. The highest
wisdom will secure the survival and propaga-
tion of the fittest. Physiology teaches that
this result, the attainment of which our hopes
prophecy, is to be secured, not by an identical education, or an identical co-education of
the sexes, but by *a special and appropriate
education, that shall produce a just and harmonious development of every part.*

Let one remark be made here. It has been
asserted that the chief reason why the higher

of age. Ten years later, there were 1,863, or 89 less children
to every thousand women than in 1830. In 1850, this number had declined to 1,720 ; in 1860, to 1,666 ; and in 1870, to
1,568. The total decline in the forty years was 384, or about
20 per cent of the whole proportional number in 1830, a generation ago. The United-States census of 1870 shows that
there is, in the city of New York, but one child under fifteen
years of age, to each thousand nubile women, when there
ought to be three ; and the same is true of our other large
cities. — *The Nation,* Aug. 28, 1873, p. 145.

and educated classes have smaller families
than the lower and uneducated is, that the
former criminally prevent or destroy increase.
The pulpit,* as well as the medical press, has
cried out against this enormity. That a disposition to do this thing exists, and is often
carried into effect, is not to be denied, and
cannot be too strongly condemned. On the
other hand, it should be proclaimed, to the
credit and honor of our cultivated women,
and as a reproach to the identical education
of the sexes, that many of them bear in
silence the accusation of self-tampering, who
are denied the oft-prayed-for trial, blessing,
and responsibility of offspring. As a matter
of personal experience, my advice has been
much more frequently and earnestly sought
by those of our best classes who desired to
know how to obtain, than by those who
wished to escape, the offices of maternity.

The experiment of the identical co-education of the sexes has been set on foot by some
of our Western colleges. It has not yet

---

* Vid. a pamphlet by the Rev. Dr. Todd.

been tried long enough to show much more than its first fruits, viz., its results while the students are in college; and of these the only obvious ones are increased emulation, and intellectual development and attainments. The defects of the reproductive mechanism, and the friction of its action, are not exhibited there; nor is there time or opportunity in college for the evils which these defects entail to be exhibited. President Magoun of Iowa College tells us, that, in the institution over which he presides, " Forty-two young men and fifty-three young ladies have pursued college courses; " and adds, " Nothing needs to be said as to the control of the two sexes in the college. The young ladies are placed under the supervision of a lady principal and assistant as to deportment, and every thing besides recitations (in which they are under the supervision of the same professors and other teachers with the young men, reciting with them); and one simple rule as to social intercourse governs every thing. The moral and religious influences attending the arrangement have been most happy." * From this it is evident that Iowa College is trying the identical co-education of the sexes ; and the president reports the happy moral and religious results of the experiment, but leaves us ignorant of its physiological results. It may never have occurred to him, that a class of a hundred young ladies might graduate from Iowa College or Antioch College or Michigan University, whose average health during their college course had appeared to the president and faculty as good as that of their male classmates who had made equal intellectual progress with them, upon whom no scandal had dropped its venom, who might be presented to the public on Commencement Day as specimens of as good health as their uneducated sisters, with roses in their cheeks as natural as those in their hands, the major part of whom might, notwithstanding all this, have physical defects that a physiologist could easily discover, and

---

* The New Englander, July, 1873. Art., Iowa College.

that would produce, sooner or later, more or
less of the sad results we have previously
described. A philanthropist and an intelligent observer, who has for a long time taken
an active part in promoting the best education of the sexes, and who still holds some
sort of official connection with a college
occupied with identical co-education, told the
writer a few months ago, that he had endeavored to trace the post-college history of the
female graduates of the institution he was
interested in. His object was to ascertain
how their physique behaved under the stress,
—the wear and tear of woman's work in
life. The conclusion that resulted from his
inquiry he formulated in the statement, that
"the co-education of the sexes is intellectually
a success, physically a failure." Another
gentleman, more closely connected with a
similar institution of education than the per-
son just referred to, has arrived at a similar
conclusion. Only a few female graduates
of colleges have consulted the writer profes-
sionally. All sought his advice two, three, or

more years after graduation; and, in all, the difficulties under which they labored could be distinctly traced to their college order of life and study, that is, to identical co-education. If physicians who are living in the neighborhood of the present residences of these graduates have been consulted by them in the same proportion with him, the inference is inevitable, that the ratio of invalidism among female college graduates is greater than even among the graduates of our common, high, and normal schools. All such observations as these, however, are only of value, at present, as indications of the drift of identical co-education, not as proofs of its physical fruits, or of their influence on mental force. Two or three generations, at least, of the female college graduates of this sort of co-education must come and go before any sufficient idea can be formed of the harvest it will yield. The physiologist dreads to see the costly experiment tried. The urgent reformer, who cares less for human suffering and human life than for the

10

trial of his theories, will regard the experiment with equanimity if not with complacency.

If, then, the identical co-education of the sexes is condemned both by physiology and experience, may it not be that their *special and appropriate co-education* would yield a better result than their special and appropriate *separate* education ? This is a most important question, and one difficult to resolve. The discussion of it must be referred to those who are engaged in the practical work of instruction, and the decision will rest with experience. Physiology advocates, as we have seen, the special and appropriate education of the sexes, and has only a single word to utter with regard to simple co-education, or juxtaposition in education.

That word is with regard to the common belief in the danger of improprieties and scandal as a part of co-education. There is some danger in this respect; but not a serious or unavoidable one. Doubtless there would be occasional lapses in a double-sexed college ;

and so there are outside of schoolhouses and seminaries of learning. Even the church and the clergy are not exempt from reproach in such things. There are sects, professing to commingle religion and love, who illustrate the dangers of juxtaposition even in things holy. " No physiologist can well doubt that the holy kiss of love in such cases owes all its warmth to the sexual feeling which consciously or unconsciously inspires it, or that the mystical union of the sexes lies very close to a union that is nowise mystical, when it does not lead to madness." * There is less, or certainly no more danger in having the sexes unite at the repasts of knowledge, than, as Plautus bluntly puts it, having he wits and she wits recline at the repasts of fashion. Isolation is more likely to breed pruriency than commingling to provoke indulgence. The virtue of the cloister and the cell scarcely deserves the name. A girl has her honor in her own keeping. If she can be trusted with

---

* Body and Mind. Op. cit., p. 85.

boys and men at the lecture-room and in church she can be trusted with them at school and in college. Jean Paul says, " To insure modesty, I would advise the education of the sexes together ; for two boys will preserve twelve girls, or two girls twelve boys, innocent amidst winks, jokes, and improprieties, merely by that instinctive sense which is the fore-runner of matured modesty. But I will guar-antee nothing in a school where girls are alone together, and still less when boys are." A certain amount of juxta-position is an advan-tage to each sex. More than a certain amount is an evil to both. Instinct and common sense can be safely left to draw the line of demar-cation. At the same time it is well to re-member that juxtaposition may be carried too far. Temptations enough beset the young, without adding to them. Let learn-ing and purity go hand in hand.

There are two considerations appertaining to this subject, which, although they do not belong to the physiology of the matter, de-serve to be mentioned in this connection.

One amounts to a practical prohibition, for the present at least, of the experiment of the special and appropriate co-education of the sexes ; and the other is an inherent difficulty in the experiment itself. The former can be removed whenever those who heartily believe in the success of the experiment choose to get rid of it ; and the latter by patient and intelligent effort.

The present practical prohibition of the experiment is the poverty of our colleges. Identical co-education can be easily tried with the existing organization of collegiate instruction. This has been tried, and is still going on in separate and double-sexed schools of all sorts, and has failed. Special and appropriate co-education requires in many ways, not in all, re-arrangement of the organization of instruction; and this will cost money and a good deal of it. Harvard College, for example, rich as it is supposed to be, whose banner, to use Mr. Higginson's illustration, is the red flag that the bulls of female reform are just now pitching into, — Harvard College could not under-

take the task of special and appropriate co-
education, in such a way as to give the two
sexes a fair chance, which means the *best*
chance, and the only chance it ought to give
or will ever give, without an endowment, additional to its present resources, of from one
to two millions of dollars; and it probably
would require the larger rather than the
smaller sum. And this I say advisedly. By
which I mean, not with the advice and con-
sent of the president and fellows of the college, but as an opinion founded on nearly
twenty years' personal acquaintance, as an
instructor in one of the departments of the
university, with the organization of instruction in it, and upon the demands which physiology teaches the special and appropriate
education of girls would make upon it. To
make boys half-girls, and girls half-boys, can
never be the legitimate function of any college. But such a result, the natural child of
identical co-education, is sure to follow the
training of a college that has not the pecuni-
ary means to prevent it. This obstacle is of

course a removable one. It is only necessary for those who wish to get it out of the way to put their hands in their pockets, and produce a couple of millions. The offer of such a sum, conditioned upon the liberal education of women, might influence even a body as soulless as the corporation of Harvard College is sometimes represented to be.

The inherent difficulty in the experiment of special and appropriate co-education is the difficulty of adjusting, in the same institution, the methods of instruction to the physiological needs of each sex; to the persistent type of one, and the periodical type of the other; to the demand for a margin in metamorphosis of tissue, beyond what study causes, for general growth in one sex, and for a larger margin in the other sex, that shall permit not only general growth, but also the construction of the reproductive apparatus. This difficulty can only be removed by patient and intelligent effort. The first step in the direction of removing it is to see plainly what errors or dangers lie in the way. These, or some of them, we have endeavored to point out. ' Nothing is so conducive to a right appreciation of the truth as a right appreciation of the error by which it is surrounded." * When we have acquired a belief of the facts concerning the identical education, the identical co-education, the appropriate education, and the appropriate co-education of the sexes, we shall be in a condition to draw just conclusions from them.

The intimate connection of mind and brain, the correlation of mental power and cerebral metamorphosis, explains and justifies the physiologist's demand, that in the education of girls, as well as of boys, the machinery and methods of instruction shall be carefully adjusted to their organization. If it were possible, they should be adjusted to the organization of each individual. None doubt the importance of age, acquirement,

---

* Use of the Ophthalmoscope. By T. C. Allbutt. Lon don. P. 5.

idiosyncrasy, and probable career in life, as factors in classification. Sex goes deeper than any or all of these. To neglect this is to neglect the chief factor of the problem. Rightly interpreted and followed, it will yield the grandest results. Disregarded, it will balk the best methods of teaching and the genius of the best teachers. Sex is not concerned with studies as such. These, for any thing that appears to the contrary physiologically, may be the same for the intellectual development of females as of males; but, as we have seen, it is largely concerned about an appropriate way of pursuing them. Girls will have a fair chance, and women the largest freedom and greatest power, now that legal hinderances are removed, and all bars let down, when they are taught to develop and are willing to respect their own organization. How to bring about this development and insure this respect, in a double-sexed college, is one of the problems of co-education.

It does not come within the scope of this

essay to speculate upon the ways — the regimen, methods of instruction, and other details of college life, — by which the inherent difficulties of co-education may be obviated. Here tentative and judicious experiment is better than speculation. It would seem to be the part of wisdom, however, to make the simplest and least costly experiment first; that is, to discard the identical separate education of girls as boys, and to ascertain what their appropriate separate education is, and what it will accomplish. Aided by the light of such an experiment, it would be comparatively easy to solve the more difficult problem of the appropriate co-education of the sexes.

It may be well to mention two or three details, which are so important that no system of *appropriate* female education, separate or mixed, can neglect them. They have been implied throughout the whole of the present discussion, but not distinctly enunciated. One is, that during the period of rapid development, that is, from fourteen

to eighteen,* a girl should not study as
many hours a day as a boy. " In most of
our schools," says a distinguished physiological authority previously quoted, " the hours
are too many for both boys and girls. From
a quarter of nine or nine, until half-past two,
is with us (Philadelphia schools for girls)
the common schooltime in private seminaries. The usual recess is twenty minutes or
half an hour, and it is not filled by enforced
exercise. In certain schools, — would it were
the rule, — ten minutes' recess is given after
every hour. To these hours, we must add
the time spent in study out of school. This,
for some reason, nearly always exceeds the
time stated by teachers to be necessary ; and
most girls between the age of thirteen and
seventeen thus expend two or three hours.

---

* Some physiologists consider that the period of growth
extends to a later age than this. Dr. Anstie fixes the limit
at twenty-five. He says, " The central nervous system is
more slow in reaching its fullest development ; and the brain,
especially, is many years later in acquiring its maximum of
organic consistency and functional power." — *Neuralgia, Op.
cit.,* by F. E. ANSTIE, p. 20.

Does any physician believe that it is good for a growing girl to be so occupied seven or eight hours a day? or that it is right for her to use her brains as long a time as the mechanic employs his muscles? But this is only a part of the evil. The multiplicity of studies, the number of teachers, — each eager to get the most he can out of his pupil, — the severer drill of our day, and the greater intensity of application demanded produce effects on the growing brain, which, in a vast number of cases, can be only disastrous. Even in girls of from fourteen to eighteen, such as crowd the normal school in Philadelphia, this sort of tension and this variety of study occasion an amount of ill-health which is sadly familiar to many physicians." *

Experience teaches that a healthy and growing boy may spend six hours of force daily upon his studies, and leave sufficient margin for physical growth. A girl cannot spend more than four, or, in occasional in-

---

* Wear and Tear. Op. cit., p. 33–4.

stances, five hours of force daily upon her studies, and leave sufficient margin for the general physical growth that she must make in common with a boy, and also for constructing a reproductive apparatus. If she puts as much force into her brain education as a boy, the brain or the special apparatus will suffer. Appropriate education and appropriate co-education must adjust their methods and regimen to this law.

Another detail is, that, during every fourth week, there should be a remission, and sometimes an intermission, of both study and exercise. Some individuals require, at that time, a complete intermission from mental and physical effort for a single day; others for two or three days; others require only a remission, and can do half work safely for two or three days, and their usual work after that. The diminished labor, which shall give Nature an opportunity to accomplish her special periodical task and growth, is a physiological necessity for all, however robust they may seem to be. The apportionment

of study and exercise to individual needs
cannot be decided by general rules, nor can
the decision of it be safely left to the pupil's
caprice or ambition.   Each case must be
decided upon its own merits.   The organization of studies and instruction must be flexi-
ble enough to admit of the periodical and
temporary absence of each pupil, without
loss of rank, or necessity of making up work,
from recitation, and exercise of all sorts. The
periodical type of woman's way of work
must be harmonized with the persistent type
of man's way of work in any successful plan
of co-education.

The keen eye and rapid hand of gain, of
what Jouffroy calls self-interest well understood, is sometimes quicker than the brain
and will of philanthropy to discern and in-
augurate reform.   An illustration of this
statement, and a practical recognition of the
physiological method of woman's work, lately
came under my observation.   There is an es-
tablishment in Boston, owned and carried on
by a man, in which ten or a dozen girls are

constantly employed. Each of them is given
and required to take a vacation of three days
every fourth week. It is scarcely necessary
to say that their sanitary condition is excep-
tionally good, and that the aggregate yearly
amount of work which the owner obtains is
greater than when persistent attendance and
labor was required. I have never heard of
any female school, public or private, in which
any such plan has been adopted ; nor is it
likely that any similar plan will be adopted
so long as the community entertain the conviction that a boy's education and a girl's
education should be the same, and that the
same means the boy's. What is known in
England as the Ten-hour Act, which Mr.
Mundella and Sir John Lubbock have recently
carried through Parliament, is a step in a
similar direction. It is an act providing for
the special protection of women against
over-work. It does not recognize, and probably was not intended to recognize, the
periodical type of woman's organization. It
is founded on the fact, however, which law

has been so slow to acknowledge, that the
male and female organization are not identical.*

This is not the place for the discussion of
these details, and therefore we will not dwell
upon them.   Our object is rather to show

---

* It is a curious commentary on the present aspect of the
" woman question " to see many who honestly advocate the
elevation and enfranchisement of woman, oppose any movement or law that recognizes Nature's fundamental distinc-
tion of sex.   There are those who insist upon the traditional
fallacy that man and woman are identical, and that the identity is confined to the man, with the energy of infatuation.
It appears from the Spectator, that Mr. and Mrs. Fawcett
strongly object to the Ten-hour Act, on the ground that it
discriminates unfairly against women as compared with
men.   Upon this the Spectator justly remarks, that the true
question for an objector to the bill to consider is not one of
abstract principle, but this : " Is the restraint proposed so
great as really to diminish the average productiveness of
woman's labor, or, by *increasing its efficacy,* to maintain its
level, or even improve it in spite of the hours lost ?   What is
the length of labor beyond which an average woman's constitution is overtaxed and deteriorated, and within which,
therefore, the law ought to keep them in spite of their relations, and sometimes in spite of themselves." — *Vid. Spectator,* London, June 14, 1873.

good and imperative reason why they should be discussed by others ; to show how faulty and pregnant of ill the education of American girls has been and is, and to demonstrate the truth, that the progress and development of the race depend upon the appropriate, and not upon the identical education of the sexes. Little good will be done in this direction, however, by any advice or argument, by whatever facts supported, or by whatever authority presented, unless the women of our country are themselves convinced of the evils that they have been educated into, and out of which they are determined to educate their daughters. They must breed in them the lofty spirit Wallenstein bade his be of : —

> " Leave now the puny wish, the girlish feeling,
> Oh, thrust it far behind thee ! Give thou proof
> Thou'rt the daughter of the Mighty, — his
> Who where he moves creates the wonderful.
> Meet and disarm necessity by choice."

SCHILLER : *The Piccolomini,* act iii. 8. (*Coleridge's Translation.*)

11

PART V.

THE EUROPEAN WAY.

"And let it appear that he doth not change his country manners for those of foreign parts, but only prick in some flowers of that he hath learned abroad into the customs of his own country." — LORD BACON.

ONE branch of the stream of travel that flows with steadily-increasing volume across the Atlantic, from the western to the eastern continent, passes from the United States, through Nova Scotia, to England. The traveller who follows this route is struck, almost as soon as he leaves the boundaries of the republic, with the difference between the physique of the inhabitants he encounters and that of those he has left behind him. The difference is most marked between the females of the two sections. The firmer

162

step, fuller chest, and ruddier cheek of the Nova-Scotian girl foretell still greater differences of color, form, and strength that England and the Continent present. These differences impressed one who passed through Nova Scotia not long ago very strongly. Her observations upon them are an excellent illustration of our subject, and they deserve to be read in this connection. Her remarks, moreover, are indirect but valuable testimony to the evils of our sort of identical education of the sexes. " Nova Scotia," she says, " is a country of gracious surprises."

" But most beautiful among her beauties, most wonderful among her wonders, are her children. During two weeks' travel in the Provinces, I have been constantly more and more impressed by their superiority in appearance, size, and health, to the children of the New-England and Middle States. In the outset of our journey, I was struck by it; along all the roadsides they looked up, boys *and girls*, fair, broad-cheeked, sturdy-legged, such as with us are seen only now and then.

I did not, however, realize at first that this was the universal law of the land, and that it pointed to something more than climate as a cause. But the first school that I saw, *en masse*, gave a st rtling impetus to the train of observation and influence into which I was unconsciously falling. It was a Sunday school in the little town of Wolfville, which lies between the Gaspereau and Cornwallis Rivers, just beyond the meadows of the Grand Pré, where lived Gabriel Lajeunesse, and Benedict Bellefontaine, and the rest of the ' simple Acadian farmers.' I arrived too early at one of the village churches ; and, while I was waiting for a sexton, a door opened, and out poured the Sunday school, whose services had just ended. On they came, dividing in the centre, and falling to the right and left about me, thirty or forty boys and girls, between the ages of seven and fifteen. They all had fair skins, red cheeks, and clear eyes ; they were all broad-shouldered, straight, and sturdy ; the younger ones were more than sturdy, — they were fat, from the ankles up.

But perhaps the most noticeable thing of all was the quiet, sturdy, unharassed expression which their faces wore ; a look which is the greatest charm of a child's face, but which we rarely see in children over two or three years old. Boys of eleven or twelve were there, with shoulders broader than the average of our boys at sixteen, and yet with the pure childlike look on their faces. Girls of ten or eleven were there, who looked almost like women, — that is, like ideal women, — simply because they looked so calm and undisturbed. . . . Out of them all there was but one child who looked sickly. He had evidently met with some accident, and was lame. Afterward, as the congregation assembled, I watched the fathers and *mothers* of these children. They, too, were broad-shouldered, tall, and straight, *especially the women.* Even old women were straight, like the negroes one sees at the South walking with burdens on their heads.

 " Five days later I saw, in Halifax, the celebration of the anniversary of the settlement of the Province. The children of the city and of some of the neighboring towns marched in ' Bands of Hope,' and processions such as we see in the cities of the States on the Fourth of July. This was just the opportunity I wanted. It was the same here as in the country. I counted, on that day, just eleven sickly-looking children ; no more! Such brilliant cheeks, such merry eyes, such evident strength, — it was a scene to kindle the dullest soul! There were scores of little ones there, whose droll, fat legs would have drawn a crowd in Central Park ; and they all had that same quiet, composed, well-balanced expression of countenance of which I spoke before, and of which it would be hard to find an instance in all Central Park.

"Climate, undoubtedly, has something to do with this. The air is moist ; and the mercury rarely rises above 80°, or falls below 10°. Also the comparative quiet of their lives helps to make them so beautiful and strong. But the most significant fact to my mind is, that, until the past year, there have been in Nova Scotia no public schools, comparatively few

private ones; and in these there is no severe
pressure brought to bear on the pupils. . . .
I must not be understood to argue from the
health of the children of Nova Scotia, as contrasted with the lack of health among our
children, that it is best to have no public
schools; only that it is better to have no public schools than to have such public schools
as are now killing off our children. . . . In
Massachusetts, the mortality from diseases of
the brain and nervous system is eleven per
cent. In Nova Scotia it is only eight per
cent." *

It would be interesting and instructive to
ascertain, if we could, the regimen of female
education in Europe. The acknowledged and
unmistakable differences between American
and European girls and women — the delicate bloom, unnatural weakness, and prema-
ture decay of the former, contrasted with the
bronzed complexion, developed form, and
enduring force of the latter — are not ade-

---

* Bits of Talk. By H. H. Pp. 71-75.

quately explained by climate. Given sufficient time, difference of climate will produce
immense differences of form, color, and force
in the same species of animals and men. But
a century does not afford a period long enough
for the production of great changes. That
length of time could not transform the sturdy
German fraulein and robust English damsel
into the fragile American miss. Everybody
recognizes and laments the change that has
been and is going on. " The race of strong,
hardy, cheerful girls, that used to grow up in
country places, and made the bright, neat,
New-England kitchens of olden times, — the
girls that could wash, iron, brew, bake, har-
ness a horse and drive him, no less than braid
straw, embroider, draw, paint, and read innumerable books, — this race of women, pride
of olden time, is daily lessening ; and, in their
stead, come the fragile, easy-fatigued, lan-
guid girls of a modern age, drilled in book-
learning, ignorant of common things." *   No

* House and Home Papers. By Harriet Beecher Stowe.
P. 205.

similar change has been wrought, during the past century, upon the mass of females in Europe. There —

> "Nature keeps the reverent frame
> With which her years began."

If we could ascertain the regimen of European female education, so as to compare it fairly with the American plan of the identical education of the sexes, it is not impossible that the comparison might teach us how it is, that conservation of female force makes a part of trans-Atlantic, and deterioration of the same force a part of cis-Atlantic civilization. It is probable such an inquiry would show that the disregard of the female organization, which is a palpable and pervading principle of American education, either does not exist at all in Europe, or exists only in a limited degree.

With the hope of obtaining information upon this point, the writer addressed inquiries to various individuals, who would be likely to have the desired knowledge. Only a few answers to his inquiries have been received up to the present writing; more are promised by and

by. The subject is a delicate and difficult
one to investigate. The reports of committees
and examining boards, of ministers of instruction, and other officials, throw little or no light
upon it. The matter belongs so much to the
domestic economy of the household and
school, that it is not easy to learn much that
is definite about it except by personal inspection and inquiry. The little information that
has been received, however, is important. It
indicates, if it does not demonstrate, an
essential difference between the regimen or
organization, using these terms in their broadest sense, of female education in America
and in Europe.

Dr. H. Hagen, an eminent physician and
naturalist of Königsburg, Prussia, now connected with the Museum of Comparative Zo-
ology at Cambridge, writes from Germany,
where he has been lately, in reply to these inquiries, as follows: —

NUREMBERG, July 23, 1873.

DEAR SIR, — The information, given by
two prominent physicians in Berlin, in an-

swer to the questions in your letter, is mostly
of a negative character. I believe them to
prove that generally girls here are doing very
well as to the catamenial function.

First, most of the girls in North Germany
begin this function in the fifteenth year, or
even later ; of course some few sooner, even
in the twelfth year or before ; but the rule is
after the fifteenth year. Now, nearly all leave
the school in the fifteenth year, and then follow some lectures given at home at leisure.
The school-girls are of course rarely troubled
by the periodical function.

There is an established kind of tradition
giving the rule for the regimen during the
catamenial period : this regimen goes from
mother to daughter, and the advice of physicians is seldom asked for with regard to it.
As a rule, the greatest care is taken to avoid
any cold or exposure at this time. If the
girls are still school-girls, they go to school,
study and write as at other times, *provided
the function is normally performed.*

School-girls never ride in Germany, nor are

they invited to parties or to dancing-parties. All this comes after the school. And even then care is taken to *stay at home when the periodical function is present.*

Concerning the health of the German girls, as compared with American girls, the German physicians have not sufficient information to warrant any statement. But the health of the German girls is commonly good except in the higher classes in the great capitals, where the same obnoxious agencies are to be found in Germany as in the whole world. But here also there is a very strong exception, or, better, a difference between America and Germany, as German girls are never accustomed to the free manners and modes of life of American girls. As a rule, in Germany, the mother directs the manner of living of the daughter entirely.

I shall have more and better information some time later.

Yours,

H. HAGEN.

A German lady, who was educated in the schools of Dantzic, Prussia, afforded information, which, as far as it went, confirmed the above. Three customs, or habits, which exert a great influence upon the health and development of girls, appear from Dr. Hagen's letter to make a part of the German female educational regimen. The first is, that girls leave school at about the age of fifteen or sixteen, that is, as soon as the epoch of rapid sexual development arrives. It appears, moreover, that during this epoch, or the greater part of it, a German girl's education is carried on at home, by means of lectures or private arrangements. These, of course, are not as inflexible as the rigid rules of a technical school, and admit of easy adjustment to the periodical demands of the female constitution. The second is the traditional motherly supervision and careful regimen of the catamenial week. Evidently the notion that a boy's education and a girl's education should be the same, and that the same means the boy s, has not yet penetrated the German mind. This has not yet evolved the idea of the identical education of the sexes. It appears that in Germany, schools, studies, parties, walks, rides, dances, and the like, are not allowed to displace or derange the demands of Nature. The female organization is respected. The third custom is, that German school-girls are not invited to parties at all. " All this comes after the school," says Dr. Hagen. The brain is not worked by day in the labor of study, and tried by night with the excitement of the ball. Pleasant recreation for children of both sexes, and abundance of it, is provided for them, all over Germany, — is regarded as necessity for them, — is made a part of their daily life ; but then it is open-air, oxygen-surrounding, blood-making, health-giving, innocent recreation ; not gas, furnaces, low necks, spinal trails, the civilized representatives of caudal appendages, and late hours.

Desirous of obtaining, if pos_ible, a more exact notion than even a physician could give of the German, traditional method of managing the catamenial function for the first few years after its appearance, I made inquiries of a German lady, now a mother, whose family name holds an honored place, both in German diplomacy and science, and who has enjoyed corresponding opportunities for an experimental acquaintance with the German regimen of female education. The following is her reply. For obvious reasons, the name of the writer is not given. She has been much in this country as well as in Germany; a fact that explains the knowledge of American customs that her letter exhibits.

My Dear Doctor, — I have great pleasure in answering your inquiries in regard to the course, which, to my knowledge, German mothers adopt with their daughters at the catamenial period. As soon as a girl attains maturity in this respect, which is seldom before the age of sixteen, she is ordered to observe complete rest; not only rest of the body, but rest of the mind. Many mothers oblige their daughters to remain in bed for three days, if they are at all delicate in health; but even those who are physically very strong are obliged to abstain from study, to remain in their rooms for three days, and keep perfectly quiet. During the whole of each period, they are not allowed to run, walk much, ride, skate, or dance. In fact, entire repose is strictly enforced in every well-regulated household and school. A German girl would consider the idea of going to a party at such times as simply preposterous; and the difference that exists in this respect in America is wholly unintelligible to them.

As a general rule, a married woman in Germany, even after she has had many children, is as strong and healthy, if not more so, than when she was a girl. In America, with a few exceptions, it appears to be the reverse; and, I have no doubt, it is owing to the want of care on the part of girls at this particular time, and to the neglect of their mothers to enforce proper rules in this most important matter.

It has seemed to me, often, that the difference in the education of girls in America and in Germany, as regards their physical training, is, that in America it is marked by a great degree of recklessness; while in Germany, the erring, if it can be called erring, is on the side of anxious, extreme caution. Therefore beautiful American girls fade rapidly ; while the German girls, who do not possess the same natural advantages, do possess, as a rule, good, permanent health, which goes hand-in-hand with happiness and enjoyment of life.

Believe me,

Very truly yours,

——— ————.

June 21, 1873.

This letter confirms the statement of Dr. Hagen, and shows that the educational and social regimen of a German school-girl is widely different from that of her American sister. Perhaps, as is intimated above, the German way, which is probably the European way also, may err on the side of too great confinement and caution; and that a medium between that and the recklessness of the American way would yield a better result than either one of them.

German peasant girls and women work in the field and shop with and like men. None who have seen their stout and brawny arms can doubt the force with which they wield the hoe and axe. I once saw, in the streets of Coblentz, a woman and a donkey yoked to the same cart, while a man, with a whip in his hand, drove the team. The by-standers did not seem to look upon the moving group as if it were an unusual spectacle. The donkey appeared to be the most intelligent and refined of the three. The sight symbolized the physical force and infamous degradation of the lower classes of women in Europe. The urgent problem of modern civilization is how to retain this force, and get rid of the degradation. Physiology declares that the solution of it will only be possible when the education of girls is made appro-

priate to their organization. A German girl,
yoked with a donkey and dragging a cart,
is an exhibition of monstrous muscular and
aborted brain development. An American
girl, yoked with a dictionary, and laboring
.he catamenia, is an exhibition of mon-
ɜ brain and aborted ovarian development.
.e investigations incident to the prepa-
n of this monograph have suggested a
ɪber of subjects kindred to the one of
.ch it treats, that ought to be discussed
m the physiological standpoint in the
terest of sound education. Some, and per-
ɪps the most important, of them are the
relation of the male organization, so far as
it is different from the female, to the labor
of education and of life ; the comparative
influence of crowding studies, that is of
excessive brain activity, upon the cerebral
metamorphosis of the two sexes; the influence of study, or brain activity, upon sleep,
and through sleep, or the want of it, upon
nutrition and development ; and, most important of all, the true relation of education to

the just and harmonious development of every part, both of the male and female organization, in which the rightful control of the cerebral ganglia over the whole system and all its functions shall be assured in each sex, and thus each be enabled to obtain the largest possible amount of intellectual and spiritual power. The discussion of these subjects at the present time would largely exceed the natural limits of this essay. They can only be suggested now, with the hope that other and abler observers may be induced to examine and discuss them.

In conclusion, let us remember that physiology confirms the hope of the race by asserting that the loftiest heights of intellectual and spiritual vision and force are free to each sex, and accessible by each ; but adds that each must climb in its own way, and accept its own limitations, and, when this is done, promises that each will find the doing of it, not to weaken or diminish, but to develop power. Physiology condemns the identical, and pleads for the appropriate education of the sexes, so that boys may become men, and girls women, and both have a fair chance to do and become their best.

Medicine & Society In America

An Arno Press/New York Times Collection

Alcott, William A. **The Physiology of Marriage.** 1866. New Introduction by Charles E. Rosenberg.

Beard, George M. **American Nervousness: Its Causes and Consequences.** 1881. New Introduction by Charles E. Rosenberg.

Beard, George M. **Sexual Neurasthenia.** 5th edition. 1898.

Beecher, Catharine E. **Letters to the People on Health and Happiness.** 1855.

Blackwell, Elizabeth. **Essays in Medical Sociology.** 1902. Two volumes in one.

Blanton, Wyndham B. **Medicine in Virginia in the Seventeenth Century.** 1930.

Bowditch, Henry I. **Public Hygiene in America.** 1877.

Bowditch, N[athaniel] I. **A History of the Massachusetts General Hospital: To August 5, 1851.** 2nd edition. 1872.

Brill, A. A. **Psychanalysis: Its Theories and Practical Application.** 1913.

Cabot, Richard C. **Social Work:** Essays on the Meeting-Ground of Doctor and Social Worker. 1919.

Cathell, D. W. **The Physician Himself and What He Should Add to His Scientific Acquirements.** 2nd edition. 1882. New Introduction by Charles E. Rosenberg.

The Cholera Bulletin. Conducted by an Association of Physicians. Vol. I: Nos. 1–24. 1832. All published. New Introduction by Charles E. Rosenberg.

Clarke, Edward H. **Sex in Education;** or, A Fair Chance for the Girls. 1873.

Committee on the Costs of Medical Care. **Medical Care for the American People:** The Final Report of The Committee on the Costs of Medical Care, No. 28. [1932].

Currie, William. **An Historical Account of the Climates and Diseases of the United States of America.** 1792.

Davenport, Charles Benedict. **Heredity in Relation to Eugenics.** 1911. New Introduction by Charles E. Rosenberg.

Davis, Michael M. **Paying Your Sickness Bills.** 1931.

Disease and Society in Provincial Massachusetts: Collected Accounts, 1736–1939. 1972.

Earle, Pliny. **The Curability of Insanity:** A Series of Studies. 1887.

Falk, I. S., C. Rufus Rorem, and Martha D. Ring. **The Costs of Medical Care:** A Summary of Investigations on The Economic Aspects of the Prevention and Care of Illness, No. 27. 1933.

Faust, Bernhard C. **Catechism of Health:** For the Use of Schools, and for Domestic Instruction. 1794.

Flexner, Abraham. **Medical Education in the United States and Canada:** A Report to The Carnegie Foundation for the Advancement of Teaching, Bulletin Number Four. 1910.

Gross, Samuel D. **Autobiography of Samuel D. Gross, M.D.,** with Sketches of His Contemporaries. Two volumes. 1887.

Hooker, Worthington. **Physician and Patient;** or, A Practical View of the Mutual Duties, Relations and Interests of the Medical Profession and the Community. 1849.

Howe, S. G. **On the Causes of Idiocy.** 1858.

Jackson, James. **A Memoir of James Jackson, Jr., M.D.** 1835.

Jennings, Samuel K. **The Married Lady's Companion, or Poor Man's Friend.** 2nd edition. 1808.

The Maternal Physician; a Treatise on the Nurture and Management of Infants, from the Birth until Two Years Old. 2nd edition. 1818. New Introduction by Charles E. Rosenberg.

Mathews, Joseph McDowell. **How to Succeed in the Practice of Medicine.** 1905.

McCready, Benjamin W. **On the Influences of Trades, Professions, and Occupations in the United States, in the Production of Disease.** 1943.

Mitchell, S. Weir. **Doctor and Patient.** 1888.

Nichols, T[homas] L. **Esoteric Anthropology: The Mysteries of Man.** [1853].

Origins of Public Health in America: Selected Essays, 1820–1855. 1972.

Osler, Sir William. **The Evolution of Modern Medicine.** 1922.

The Physician and Child-Rearing: Two Guides, 1809–1894. 1972.

Rosen, George. **The Specialization of Medicine:** with Particular Reference to Ophthalmology. 1944.

Royce, Samuel. **Deterioration and Race Education.** 1878.

Rush, Benjamin. **Medical Inquiries and Observations.** Four volumes in two. 4th edition. 1815.

Shattuck, Lemuel, Nathaniel P. Banks, Jr., and Jehiel Abbott. **Report of a General Plan for the Promotion of Public and Personal Health.** Massachusetts Sanitary Commission. 1850.

Smith, Stephen. **Doctor in Medicine** and Other Papers on Professional Subjects. 1872.

Still, Andrew T. **Autobiography of Andrew T. Still,** with a History of the Discovery and Development of the Science of Osteopathy. 1897.

Storer, Horatio Robinson. **The Causation, Course, and Treatment of Reflex Insanity in Women.** 1871.

Sydenstricker, Edgar. **Health and Environment.** 1933.

Thomson, Samuel. **A Narrative, of the Life and Medical Discoveries of Samuel Thomson.** 1822.

Ticknor, Caleb. **The Philosophy of Living;** or, The Way to Enjoy Life and Its Comforts. 1836.

U.S. Sanitary Commission. **The Sanitary Commission of the United States Army:** A Succinct Narrative of Its Works and Purposes. 1864.

White, William A. **The Principles of Mental Hygiene.** 1917.